PERSPECTIVES ON HEALTH COMMUNICATION

Barbara C. Thornton
University of Nevada, Reno

Gary L. Kreps
Northern Illinois University

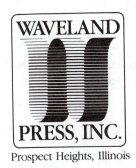

WAVELAND

PRESS, INC.

Prospect Heights, Illinois

For information about this book, write or call:

Waveland Press, Inc.
P.O. Box 400
Prospect Heights, Illinois 60070
(708) 634-0081

Consulting Editor

Robert E. Denton, Jr.

Contents

CHAPTER 8

Ethical Communication in Health Care   179

CHAPTER 9

Communication and Health Promotion   205

Preface

The readings in this book were selected to stimulate thought about the central role of communication in health and health care. They are certainly not exhaustive of all areas of health communication inquiry and practice, but do cover most major health communication topics. The readings were chosen because they are provocative and represent different health care consumer and provider perspectives on health communication. We hope they will be excellent discussion starters for classes and training groups, enabling students, health care providers, and consumers to examine relevant health communication issues.

We invited several esteemed colleagues, Deborah Ballard-Reisch, Lee Ann Glass, Greg Hayes, Trudy Larson, Edward Maibach, Rosalie Martinelli, and Dorothy Rasinski to prepare original readings for the book. We included seminal readings from other esteemed colleagues including Dean Barnlund, Eileen Berlin Ray, June Flora, Katherine Miller, Joe Turow and Seymour Shubin. We appreciate the work of the many authors whose work we showcase in this book of readings. We included several of our own readings in this book. We hope you will enjoy these readings and that they will also enhance your understanding of health communication.

As a collection of the expertise of several authors, this book of readings reflects different styles, formats and footnotes. In order to preserve the integrity of the writings, we chose not to alter the readings. Even the language of the authors reflects differing viewpoints. For example, several authors have chosen to use the more traditional word "patient" instead of "client," or "health care" instead of "healthcare."

This book can be utilized by itself or can accompany a text such as the one designed as complementary to this reader: *Health Communication: Theory and Practice, Second Edition* by Gary L. Kreps and Barbara C. Thornton. If the latter book is chosen to accompany this reader, it should be noted that the readings are designed to follow each of the chapters. We also encourage the use of this reader by itself or with other texts or articles designed to study health communication or a related field.

We thank Neil and Carol Rowe of Waveland Press for their support and encouragement in producing this book, and we express our appreciation to Laurie Albright for assisting with the editing process. We also appreciate the endurance of our families. We dedicate this book to Dan Thornton for his courageous behavior and optimism as he recovered from a near-fatal accident as this book was being edited.

CHAPTER

1

Communication in Health Care

Human communication performs a central role in the delivery of health care and the promotion of health. Health care providers depend on their abilities to communicate effectively with clients and co-workers to gather pertinent information for guiding health care activities and eliciting cooperation in the provision of health care. Health care consumers also depend on communication to make their health care needs known and for gathering relevant health information to direct their own health care. Unfortunately, a large body of literature clearly indicates that communication in health care is often ineffective, leading to problems such as miscommunication, misinformation, dehumanization, insensitive interactions, dissatisfaction, and a lack of cooperation between interdependent health care providers and consumers (see Kreps & Thornton, 1992). This book of readings is designed to provide health care providers and consumers with a heightened awareness of the importance of communication in health care and strategies for communicating effectively in health care situations by illustrating the complexities and subtleties of health communication.

1

The two readings in this section of the book examine the role of communication in health care from the perspectives of both health care providers and health care consumers.

The first reading, "A Model For Interdisciplinary Learning In Health Care," was written specifically for this book by a group of faculty members from the Department of Community Health Sciences of the University of Nevada, Reno. The reading critiques current models of education for health care professionals and presents an alternative curricular model that identifies four interdependent areas for study: personal, interpersonal/small group, scientific/technical, and community/global, all incorporating health communication and interdisciplinary education. They contend that a balanced educational perspective, like the one they present, can effectively prepare health professionals to meet the health care system demands of the future.

The second reading, "Offer Families Hope . . . Or Help Them Let Go," describes a real health care case originally presented at a Nursing Grand Rounds (group review of cases) at the University of Kentucky Hospital in Lexington. It is written by Seymour Shubin. The case is about Anna, a young woman who received severe brain injuries in a car accident, her treatment, and her family's responses to her treatment. After her case is described, her father's account is presented, followed by the nurses' perspective on the case. This reading provides a powerful testimony to the importance of sharing information and feelings in health care on the part of both family members and health care providers. It clearly illustrates the complexities and ambiguities of modern health care, as well as how misperceptions and false hopes can influence health communication. Many of the issues suggested in this reading (informed consent, bioethics committees, honesty, social support, health care decision making, hospital policies and bureaucracy) are examined in greater depth in Kreps and Thornton's *Health Communication: Theory and Practice, Second Edition* (1992).

Kreps, G. L. & Thornton, B. C. (1992). *Health Communication: Theory and Practice* 2nd edition. Prospect Heights, IL: Waveland Press.

1

A Model for Interdisciplinary Learning in Health Care

By *Barbara C. Thornton, Rosalie D. Marinelli,*
and *Gregory Hayes*

Few dispute that the nation is in a health care crisis especially in rural areas and the inner cities (Colloton, 1989). While the crisis is multi-faceted, contributing factors to the present situation may be the education and selection processes that attract science and technology-oriented individuals to the health professions. Social and behavioral training are minimal. These factors form the basis of many of today's medical problems. Until we address these problems by changing the focus of professional education, we will find it difficult to make major strides in responding to the current crisis (Clawson, 1990; Rogers, 1988; Ebert & Ginzberg, 1988; Burg, et al., 1988; Leslie, et al., 1988; Givner, 1986; McCue, 1985; Vaux, 1985; GPEP Report, 1984).

Most medical and dental students complete four or more years of college preparation, as do many other preprofessionals. The rationale for a college education of this length has been that a health care provider should be broadly educated in the humanities and sciences before embarking upon professional studies. However, a look at the course requirements that prepare a student to apply to professional schools indicates the students spend an inordinate amount of time on natural sciences and mathematics with much less emphasis placed on the humanities (Clawson, 1990; GPEP, 1984).

We are suggesting that preprofessional students be given the opportunity to choose a series of courses that complement any major and allow a broader experience integrating the social, behavioral and natural sciences with the humanities. We have analyzed the qualities and skills which have been suggested in the literature for the future health care professional and have

This article was written especially for this collection. The authors are members of the faculty in the Department of Community Health Sciences, College of Human and Community Sciences, University of Nevada, Reno.

divided them into four zones: (1) personal, (2) interpersonal/small group, (3) scientific/technical, (4) community/global. We propose that students entering professional schools in the future should have training and understanding in these four areas and we will suggest a model, already being tested, that promotes this position. Figure 1 demonstrates the zones and components of our model.

Figure 1

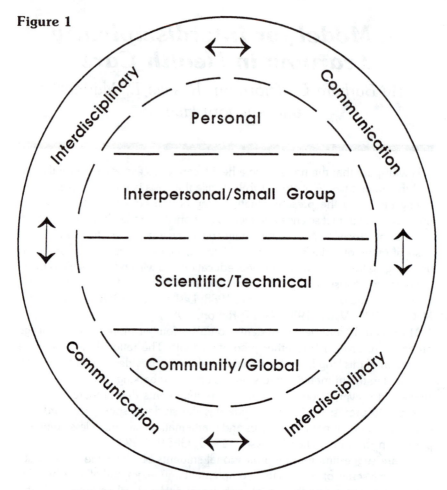

**Education Zones for Health Professional
Education in the 21st Century**

The use of the word zone is deliberate. "Zone" indicates a permeable area with particular features, properties, purposes and uses. These zones, necessary to the health professional of the future, are continually over-lapping and should not be isolated one from the other.

Educational Zones for the Health Professional

We use this symbolic model since it is our view and the view of the educators cited previously that the challenges of the twenty-first century will be more globally oriented. The future will demand that the health care provider have the capacity to discern issues yet unknown. Professional education requires not only an understanding of the world but also the imagination to shape that world (Weldon, 1987). We will discuss these zones and the educational strategy related to each area. The importance of communication and an interdisciplinary approach is acknowledged throughout each zone.

1. The Personal Zone

This educational zone is one in which introspective skills and responsibilities are developed. Physical, mental and spiritual issues are of particular importance in developing the personal zone of the helping professional in order to strengthen the attributes necessary for clear thinking and decision making as well as personal development and ethical leadership (Jonsen, 1987). An emphasis on these skills is advocated by all major medical professional organizations. Personal health and lifestyles, insight into one's personal values and the interdisciplinary study of ethics are important in this area. Communication is emphasized because it is the translating mechanism whereby theory becomes practice.

2. The Interpersonal/Small Group Zone

In this area, the student develops skills and insight into working both with others (such as clients and colleagues) in one-to-one interaction and with small groups related to health care (such as ethics committees and community advisory boards). Communication skills are also important in this zone. These skills include such areas as conflict resolution, reflective listening and leadership. Interpersonal and small group dynamics have future application for doctor-patient relationships and health care team leaders. For example, a recent American Dental Association survey indicates the practice of dentistry is undergoing a dramatic shift in focus to health care teams. This follows the trend being established in other health professions. A focus on teams is a result of the increasing size of practices using more staff and auxiliary help as well as the attraction of young professionals to non-solo practice modalities. Yet many faculty admit that schools do a poor job in preparing professionals to manage their practices and staff, to work collaboratively and to communicate effectively with their colleagues (Koldenberg, Becker and Hallan, 1990).

The increase in the elderly and disabled population is an example of one such demographic change that will demand the team approach.

3. The Scientific/Technical Zone

In order to solve problems, be they individual or global, the health professional of the twenty-first century will need to be well trained and knowledgeable in mathematics, the use of computers and the natural sciences in order to evaluate clinical problems, conduct research and apply knowledge appropriately. Whereas this zone has been overemphasized in the education of professionals in the twentieth century, it should not be minimized in the twenty-first. Overemphasis is a problem only in the sense that other equally important areas of learning and development have been generally ignored. What is needed for the future is a more balanced and integrated approach which acknowledges the full breadth of training necessary to produce the very best health care providers and a reevaluation of the specific courses that will achieve this goal (GPEP Report, 1984; Bishop, 1984).

4. The Community/Global Zone

Learning to analyze, critically evaluate and solve community health problems and problems of global importance are vital to the education of the future health professional. Whether the issues are pollution or diseases such as AIDS, the health care provider needs the skills to understand and to influence thoughtful and responsible long-range policy. This community responsibility mandates the need to integrate basic science material and increasing amounts of social and behavioral sciences, ethics and health policy. The importance of appreciating cultural diversity, such as age, race or gender is important in all four zones but particularly in this area.

Current Educational Model

At the University of Nevada, Reno in the Department of Community Health Sciences, we have been developing and implementing over the past fourteen years an educational model which incorporates the four zones discussed; it responds to the neglected facets of student development and maintains the traditional requirements in science and mathematics.

The core courses of this new model focus on issues in both the natural and social sciences plus the humanities with examples from the health care field. This kind of teaching allows individuals the opportunity to:

1. examine their decision to enter health care by determining their level of comfort with the realities of the health sphere.
2. be exposed to the literature and vocabulary of bioethics, interpersonal dynamics, public policy and health education, and
3. develop their level of social awareness and individual responsibility.

These goals are met by offering core courses in personal health, communication skills and interpersonal dynamics, bioethics, health education and health policy. Community fieldwork experiences are required and intensive advisement is continuous throughout the student's baccalaureate process.

Emphasis on personal health, lifestyle choices and ethical issues assists students to, first and foremost, gain insight into themselves. This is accomplished by helping them examine the dramatic effect of their personal choices on the quality of their health, as well as the health of others. Insight into values and priorities yields an ability to be cognizant of personal beliefs and biases and, thus, to approach difficult issues with clearer vision.

Development at a personal level leads naturally to the powerful need to communicate more effectively and honestly with others — to express thoughts, feelings and, more importantly, to listen and reflect on other points of view. Pivotal courses in communication skills and ethical issues in health care help students to develop their abilities to communicate, to set aside biases as much as possible, to listen well, to analyze carefully and critically all the points of view expressed, to determine the best course of action by the group and, consensus or not, to recognize the critical need to act even in the absence of the "right" answer. The use of the case study method in small groups in such courses as ethics and communication encourages participation in a non-judgmental environment and teaches interpersonal and small group skills.

The small group setting also provides an important opportunity to develop leadership ability and peer learning. Leaders for the ethics and communication skills courses are chosen from the most thoughtful, perceptive, and enthusiastic students in previous classes. As leaders, these students study and discuss many of the important issues of group dynamics as well as the potential solutions to roadblocks that may arise within the group setting. Leaders are required, depending on the class, to keep diaries or complete frequent evaluation forms relating to their experiences, their goals for the group, their reactions to the group, their analysis of how best to solve problems within the group, and how these strategies for improvement actually work.

In addition to such classes as ethics and communication skills, an emphasis on fieldwork placements in a wide array of health care settings also provides an opportunity to use and develop the ethical insights and decision-making strategies learned in the classroom.

Scientific and technical knowledge is not neglected. Students complete the many biology, chemistry, physics, mathematics and psychology requirements typical of most prehealth professional majors.

One of the strengths of our model is the deliberate attempt to bridge technical and scientific learning with ethical and policy implications. For example, epidemiology draws from the scientific research with a particular focus on the social impact of illness and disease, combining empirical information with behavioral responses and interventions. Required courses are supplemented by electives such as gerontology and drug and alcohol abuse. All strongly support the notion that the future of health care requires a team approach.

The complexity of problems facing health care in the twenty-first century are problems which often do not have a single answer, but require a very broad orientation with multidisciplinary approaches. As always, the emphasis is on communication. Bringing multiple disciplines together is not enough. Health care providers must also listen to and work with each other, recognizing their diverse backgrounds and the multitude of agendas, values and priorities that affect the choices they make. Regardless of discipline or profession, the importance of working collaboratively on a broad spectrum of issues from client intervention to community concerns is essential (Warren, 1985). In order to promote this effort, students need to have an appreciation of the roles and contributions of other disciplines. Experience in developing trust is enhanced by having worked together in classroom and clinical settings. Collaborative efforts such as we suggest will take leadership. Traditionally physicians and dentists have been leaders in actual practice but because of the changing client profile from acute to chronic care, it is now common to find team leaders from a variety of disciplines. As the environment for the delivery of health services changes, not only must the future practitioner come to terms with these developments but so must the educational programs that prepare them.

The use of a team approach emphasizes interdependence among members, enhances collaborative efforts and promotes consensus leadership (Wharton, 1987). Demographic changes not only impact doctors but also physical therapists, occupational therapists, pharmacists and other professionals necessary in long-term and rehabilitative care. Issues in health policy likewise draw on an array of disciplines in the quest for answers. Students in policy classes debate the most important issues in health care today: access to care, quality of care, cost containment, rationing of resources, the role of competition, the problems of the uninsured, the changing role of physicians and so on. Students also study a variety of other health care systems to gain a greater understanding of how these systems respond to similar problems. Such a focus leads to an appreciation of the community and global nature of modern health care problems.

A community or global focus encourages students to step back and see the "big picture," to understand that the effects of health problems are not just on individuals but on whole populations — ethnic groups, risk groups, communities, societies. They learn to recognize that problems in health care often transcend the traditional boundaries of the medical office or the hospital and that some are so broad as to be truly worldwide in scope.

Our experience with this model, based on the four zones (personal, interpersonal/small group, scientific/technical and community/global), indicates to us that this kind of education should not be limited to the undergraduate programs but should be continued throughout the professional education process. Students who have gone through the process and graduated from the program affirm our findings.

Health care professionals of tomorrow can be better educated, more well-rounded and better able to respond to the increasing demands of future health care systems if they have had the opportunity to learn more about themselves, the other disciplines with which they will work, the community and global nature of so many of the problems they will confront, and, most importantly, how to communicate effectively.

Bibliography

Bishop, J. (1984). Infuriating tensions: Science and the medical student. *Journal of Medical Education*, 59, 91-101.

Burg, F., Croll, S., Ruff, G., and Stemmier, E. (1988). Competency requirements: A new approach to medical school admissions. *JAMA*, 259, 389-391.

Clawson, D. (1990). The education of the physician. *Academic Medicine*, 65, 84-88.

Colloton, J. (1989). Academic medicine's changing covenant with society. *Academic Medicine*, 64, 55-60.

Ebert, R. and Ginzberg, E. (1988). The reform of medical education. *Health Affairs, Supplement*, 7, 5-38.

Givner, N. (1986). Cognitive and noncognitive characteristics of medical school applicants. *The Advisor*, 6, 4-5.

GPEP Report (1984). *Physicians for the Twenty-First Century*, Association of American Medical Colleges.

Jonsen, A. (1987). Leadership in meeting ethical challenges. *Journal of Medical Education*, 62, 95-99.

Koldenberg, D. Becker, B. and Hallan, J. (1990). Dentistry in the year 2000: Assessments from a Delphi panel. *Journal of the American College of Dentists*, 57.

Leslie, C., Drew, L., Chuck, E., and Horowitz, M. (1988). Making doctors human. *The Advisor*, 8, 14-15.

McCue, J. (1985). Influence of medical and premedical education on important personal qualities of physicians. *The American Journal of Medicine*, 78, 985-91.

Rogers, D. (1988). Clinical education and the doctor of tomorrow. Adapting clinical medical education to the needs of today and tomorrow. Proceedings of the Josiah Macy, Jr. Foundation. National Seminar on Medical Education. New York: New York Academy.

Vaux, K. (1985). Ethics and the future of health professions. *The Advisor*, 5, 13-15.

Warren, J. (1985). Thoughts on listening to a conference on medical education for the 21st Century. *The Advisor*, 5, 20-23.

Weldon, V. (1987). Why the dinosaurs died: Extinction or evolution. *Journal of Medical Education*, 62, 109-15.

Wharton, C.R. (1987). Leadership in medical education: the challenge of diversity. *Journal of Medical Education* 62(2), 86-94.

2

Offer Families Hope . . . or Help Them Let Go?

By *Seymour Shubin*

That day, everything was looking up for Anna. Recently promoted, she'd been busy planning her wedding, 3 weeks away. Then, driving down a winding country road to pick up her fiancé at work, she had a car accident.

Rescue workers freed her from the tangled metal and transported her by helicopter to the emergency department. She had multiple injuries: a severe closed head injury, a left hemothorax, right pneumothorax, hepatic bilateral clavical fractures, multiple rib fractures, and pulmonary and cardiac contusions. She was rushed to the operating room for liver surgery.

In the postanesthesia room, she was coded three times. After 6 hours, she was admitted to the intensive care unit (ICU). She had no evidence of brain function.

Anna had told her family in the past that she wouldn't want her life to be artificially maintained, and she'd signed an organ-donor form. But now it seemed her family wouldn't have to confront the question of prolonging her life. They were told she wouldn't live.

After her family left, however, an electroencephalogram was done, and it showed slight diffuse slowing — Anna did have brain activity and so didn't meet the criteria for brain death. In the next few hours, she began to cough and gag a little. She also had motor response to pain. The family was then called and told that she was probably going to survive.

But Anna didn't improve neurologically in the days that followed, which caused her family a lot of anxiety. To help relieve their distress, the primary nurse on the ICU got them involved in Anna's care. She told them to talk to Anna and to touch her; she taught them how to move her body in passive range-of-motion exercises. She suggested they bring in a cassette player with earphones so Anna could listen to her favorite music or recordings the family

Reprinted with permission from *Nursing90*, Vol. 20, March 1990: 44-49. Mr. Shubin is a contributing editor to *Nursing90*.

made for her. On the day Anna was transferred to the medical unit, almost 3 weeks after the accident, she turned 22. It was to have been her wedding day.

Anna's family visited her faithfully, continuing the stimulation program the primary nurse on the ICU had started. They also made a giant calendar and wrote on it any signs of improvement they perceived, such as "squeezed hand on command."

But Anna didn't improve. Later, toward the end of her stay, her father posted a copy of her hospital bill on the wall of her room. It listed everything that had been done for her, such as computed tomography scans, X-rays, and consults — and the cost. The unspoken message: "Look at all that's been done and what has changed? What's the point?"

Despite their frustration, her family decided that when Anna was ready for discharge, they'd admit her to a rehabilitation facility that did extensive work with coma patients.

Then, in the year after Anna's discharge, they decided that because her condition remained unchanged, "supportive care only" would be best for her. When Anna contracted pneumonia, she wasn't given antibiotics or transferred from the nursing facility to a hospital. About 18 months after the accident, she died.

The Father's View

By F. W. Kephart

During the first 12 hours after our daughter's accident, our only information came from the trauma doctors. They described very clearly the extensive physical injuries and the suspected severity of the brain damage. We knew nothing about brain injury, so when we asked the doctors how extensive the damage was, we were surprised to hear them say, "We don't know." We were bewildered that they couldn't "see" the injuries with some kind of technology and make a diagnosis based on their observations.

While the nurses and doctors worked to save Anna, we were desperately trying to understand the flood of words, images, and emotions that had poured in on us since the accident. The nurses and doctors were alert, objective, and professional. We, however, were numbed by shock and personal pain. All we had was our love for Anna and for one another.

How that love helped during the hours Anna was in the postanesthesia room and the ICU. We raged, cried, kicked the walls. We struggled with ourselves and with one another. We prayed, we held on to each other — and we discovered bits of peace.

We were probably as prepared as anyone could be when, about 24 hours after the accident, a doctor told us Anna wasn't going to survive.

A nurse, after carefully describing how Anna looked, invited us to come into the ICU and see her. Most of us chose not to, preferring to remember her as she'd been in life. We were then left alone — parents, brothers, sister, fiancé — like a tiny knot of survivors in an alien land. We cried a lot, but we laughed too, sharing memories. Anna was dying, and somehow it was all right.

A representative of the hospital's organ-donor program approached us, proposing that Anna be a donor. Knowing she would have wanted this, we signed — with more tears but with great pride — the permission documents.

The ICU nurses came to us then and gently encouraged us to go home and rest. We understood that our daughter's body was being kept alive so her organs could be surgically removed the next day. At home, we phoned our church and scheduled a vigil and memorial service. We contacted the funeral home and arranged for cremation. We prepared a notice for the local paper.

Different news

The next day when we phoned the hospital, however, we learned that Anna's electroencephalogram was "not consistent with brain death." We were, to say the least, amazed. We had prepared for death — not life.

Our church friends, the funeral director, and others were bewildered when we canceled the plans. This change had created a strange emotional vacuum: What could they say? What could we say?

We sensed this same dilemma when we arrived at the hospital that day. What could the doctors and nurses say to us? What could we say to them? And that's when another tragedy began.

The doctors were clearly uncomfortable. At a family conference 2 days after the accident, the staff presented two prospects — Anna might die, Anna might live. When we asked, "How long?" the doctor answered, "I don't know." When we asked, "What will her condition be?" the answer was, "We can only wait and see."

The answers were accurate, but cautious and laced with vague conditions. The doctors and nurses must have been aware, because of statistical studies and their own experiences and observations, that this was probably a case of neocortical death. But they hedged: "We just never know in cases like this."

We, on the other hand, had no experiences whatsoever to call upon, no statistics. This not only was our first child to be in such an accident, but it was also our first time on the ICU. We pressured the staff to be specific — and were finally told that the *best* result of their efforts would leave Anna needing institutional care for the rest of her life.

We knew that Anna had dreaded such a life, and later we pointedly asked a doctor if there were alternatives. He was extremely hesitant, but did cautiously mention withholding medication or nutrition. This was the only time during Anna's months in the acute care hospital that there was even a hint of an option.

That evening, we made a decision for Anna: If she coded again, she was not to be resuscitated. We phoned the hospital and asked that our request be entered on her chart.

Trying to help

At first, we felt like intruders on the ICU. We were intimidated by the technology. We felt so little, so insignificant. We'd look into the nurses' faces, seeking answers for questions we couldn't even express. When a doctor or nurse appeared, the only questions we could come up with were "How is she doing today?" or "Has she opened her eyes yet?"

And we didn't know what to say when we talked with our daughter's soul, residing in that unresponsive body. If our voices and touches were reaching her at all, what message should we give — "Hold on, babe" or "Let go, sweetheart?"

Can you imagine how we felt when one day the nurses told us that Anna's intracranial pressure dropped each time we talked to her? Finally, we were making a difference.

The nurses did talk to us a lot about hope. They said that we shouldn't lose it, that we should hold on to it. They seemed to drill this into us, insisting, "Your job is to hope. . . ."

They also barraged us with inspiring anecdotes. Every nurse we met seemed to have a story that began, "I had a patient once who was much worse than Anna . . ." and would invariably end with something miraculous like ". . . and she's home now with her family. We just never know in cases like this."

We wanted to believe the nurses, but these stories obviously conflicted with other messages we were getting. And we couldn't confront the nurses ("What is the truth? Tell us the truth!") because we needed them. How could we risk offending them when they showed such empathy, such concern? They'd become a part of our family because they shared our suffering.

The pattern that was started on the ICU continued when Anna was transferred to the medical floor. Each new procedure that was proposed by the doctor was accompanied by a form, stating goals and measurements, that we were to sign. Today, I question the notion of "informed consent" — how little "informed" someone in stress can feel — but at the time I signed anything put before me.

Our close relationship with nurses continued throughout the months that followed, as we took our daughter to specialized rehabilitation facilities. We kept searching at first for a key that would unlock her being — then finally for the key that would free her from her prison here on earth.

At each facility it was the same: nurses encouraging us to hope, doctors saying, "Yes, there's still a chance she may emerge," then hurrying off. (It was always the nurses who stayed, listening.) One doctor even said, "Oh, there's no doubt she's vegetative, but of course there's nothing we can do about that. . . ."

The final rehabilitation center was hundreds of miles from our home. Again, though far away, the nurses there were like members of our family. Although we could visit Anna only every 3 months or so, we were comforted by the feeling that the nurses' hands were as our hands; their comforting voices, echoes of ours.

Peace, at last

Eighteen months after her accident, our daughter's body died. This came about only because of our efforts to take charge of her situation. We studied and consulted with independent specialists throughout the country and concluded that she wasn't in a coma, as we'd been told, but was in a persistent vegetative state (PVS). (How I hated that term.)

With legal counsel and the cautious cooperation of the rehabilitation facility administration, we prepared special orders: Besides being considered a no-code, our daughter was not to be given antibiotics or to be transferred to an acute care hospital.

We actually participated in "training sessions" for the rehabilitation nurses and other staff to help them unlearn some things about sustaining life at any cost. And when symptoms of pneumonia appeared on the morning of March 30, 1988, the nurses followed the special orders to the letter. Anna's death was quiet and beautiful. The final curtain, at last.

Questions for the nurses

Looking back, I'm comforted by memories of all the people who held on to us during those long months. I'm grateful for — and humbled by — the profound experience.

I also look back with a sense that something was wrong, that we were victimized somehow, and that nothing has been learned. I look back with anger — not the burning anger I once had, but anger just the same.

I'd like to ask the following questions of those who cared for Anna:

- Why wasn't there a functioning medical-ethics committee at the acute care hospital to help analyze the complex dimensions of our daughter's case and to guide the staff and family?

- Why wasn't the family told of the probability of PVS or neocortical death at some time during those first weeks? She was far more than "in a coma" — a fact that was shared with all *but* the family.

- Were we, by our constant concern for our daughter and our daily presence, sending the message that we were out of touch with reality, that we didn't want to hear anything negative about Anna's condition?

- What of Anna's own stated desire regarding her body? Doctors and nurses knew from the first night that she'd signed an organ-donor card and had specifically stated that she didn't want to be artificially sustained with wires and tubes. This — along with our authorization to remove her organs — was a pretty clear message. Why wasn't it heard?

- Didn't you recognize our acceptance when you initially told us Anna would die? Didn't you hear us or learn from us then?

- Were the doctors and nurses really looking to us for guidance all the time? Did you actually want *us* to tell you what to do?

- Didn't you "hear" us wishing she could die? As parents we couldn't verbalize this; we didn't have words for such unnatural thoughts, but *yes, we wanted her to die*. Every hour we were there during the 3 months in the hospital, we wanted it to end for her and for us. We can say it aloud now, but we were saying it then, too. You must have sensed this — we were so close. But maybe not.

What should have been done?

In my opinion, a series of formal family conferences should have been set up by the hospital, under the guidance of a medical-ethics committee. The purposes would have been:

- to help the family, as decision makers, fully understand the implications of the patient's condition. This would take many hours. If the attending doctors can't or won't handle this essential task, then the hospital should hire specialists to do it. *This responsibility must not be dumped on the nurses.*

- to aid the family in considering options. Telling the family, "You need to go find a nursing home" isn't enough; yet it was the only direction offered to us. Nor is providing a list of rehabilitation facilities or a medical-journal article on withdrawal of medications enough. In cases like Anna's, expecting nurses and a social worker to inform and guide the family is unrealistic.

I wish we'd been helped to consider at least three options for Anna — to take her to a local nursing home, to get her into a "coma management" program, or to let her body die. The last is obviously the most difficult option. But how I wish we'd been given it.

Of course, everyone wanted the best for Anna and us. I suggest that we (doctors, nurses, and family) were all trapped in some way — trapped in the system — and so together we sustained Anna's suffering and humiliating imprisonment.

I think most nurses know they're in a kind of trap. You enter a profession to help people, you want to be sensitive and caring, then you find that if you're to be truthful to them — and to yourself — you sometimes have to cause them emotional pain. I say that if you ever have to choose between telling the truth and offering hope, choose truth.

Hope isn't a commodity, something that can simply be given like a pill or an injection. Patients and families get very confused when nurses talk about hope because we tend to translate it in terms of *medical* outcomes alone.

I say give us facts and probabilities; hope will take care of itself. Tell us the truth and stand with us and give us hugs now and then. Hope will find us.

Our solace now

The only solace my family and I can draw from our experience is that perhaps others will benefit from it. There are thousands of PVS victims, loving families, caring nurses, and concerned doctors entangled in this complex medical, moral, and legal web.

Help is needed on many levels, from setting up standards for early diagnosis to guidelines for terminating life support. But there can be no progress until the issues are brought before the public.

The nurses whose article accompanies this have been through the ordeal with us. Together, we take the step of identifying some of those issues and conflicts. It's a comfort to know this is a beginning.

The Nurses' View

Before presenting our perspective of Anna's care, we first want to express our admiration for the sensitive, articulate way her father has shared this ordeal — and for his many insights. Reopening painful wounds to change the system takes great courage and caring. Now that technologic advances are outstripping our capacity to deal with ethical issues, our system certainly needs drastic change.

We want to say, too, that though our perspective of Anna's case often differs from her father's, this isn't a debate in which one wins and the other loses. There's more than one truth in every experience. And so we join with him in the hope that an understanding of both perspectives will be of help to other families, other nurses.

The most obvious discrepancy between our perspectives concerns how much information Anna's family was given about her prognosis. Her father says that the hospital staff was aware that Anna was in a PVS but didn't convey this to the family.

We remember, however, that the family was repeatedly told of the possibility that Anna would never regain significant mental function. And one of us recalls a doctor on the trauma service telling the family at a very early stage that Anna would probably have to be in a nursing home for the rest of her life.

We don't know why Mr. Kephart's perception is that he wasn't told the truth early on about Anna's condition as we knew it. But we realize that many families use a coping mechanism ("minimization") in the initial stages of a serious illness that protects them from facing the brutal realities.

Anna's father is absolutely right, though, when he says that the family received mixed messages about the prognosis. He didn't mention this example, but in an early conference, the neurosurgeon, referring to various statistics, indicated that Anna might be walking and talking within a year. And nurses did say they'd seen patients as seriously injured as Anna who did get better — because they *have*.

Unfortunately, the way a patient responds to brain injury is still a mystery — and our powers of prediction often prove fallible. Sometimes we ourselves question the ethics of super-technology "rescues" of patients we'd swear would never truly live again — and then are amazed when these patients visit us later. The plain truth is that none of the staff *knew* what the outcome would be. By definition, a persistent vegetative state becomes apparent only after it's been persistent. Very likely we erred on the side of presenting a positive outcome — because that's what *we* wanted. That may have been our own coping mechanism. In any event, we weren't deliberately masking the truth.

Offering hope

Anna's father brings up another, equally complex issue — the matter of offering hope. As someone whose hopes were crushed, he urges us not to talk to families in terms of hope; instead, that we give "facts and probabilities."

If only things were that clear-cut in the world we work in day after day. Not only do our *hearts* tell us to give hope when we can, but research indicates that families of critically ill patients *need* hope. In fact, some families react angrily when we suggest that their loved one might not survive — sometimes insisting that we tell them of miraculous cures even as we're trying to prepare them for the worst.

Perhaps nurses do have an incomplete understanding of what supporting the family's hope means. But who knows which family needs hope the way it needs any other sustenance? What those of us who cared for Anna do know now is that we were wrong in our interpretation of her family's needs and thinking.

For instance, we interpreted the calendar they made, listing what they considered signs of improvement, as evidence that they were as fixed as we were on the hope that she'd improve. We made another mistake in not questioning the meaning of their behaviors. When they came in to visit every day with bright smiles, laughter, and jokes, insisting that keeping a positive attitude was going to do more for Anna than anything else, we felt they wouldn't listen to anything negative. We didn't see that they were as mentally prepared for her death — or continued existence with no change in her condition — as any family in that situation could be.

Certainly, we should never have "barraged" them with stories of miraculous recoveries. If we feel the need to preach about the importance of hope, we'd do well to look into ourselves for the reason. Do we want to hang on to hope for our own sakes?

How do we effectively pass on some realistic sense of hope to the family? Anna's father offers us, so eloquently, a key: "Tell us the truth and stand with us and give us hugs now and then. Hope will find us."

Perhaps we can also offer hope by conveying to families — through such things as they way we touch the patient and try to communicate with her amid all the tubes and wires — a feeling of her importance to us as an *individual* and as a member of that family.

Other options

What made Anna's tragedy even greater was the misunderstanding between family and staff, not only about the outcome — but also about treatment options.

The family was so quick to agree when we gave them consent-to-treat forms that we believed they knew they had options but chose to continue intensive treatment. Anna's father says now that they preferred that she die rather than linger on hopelessly — but that they were unable to put this into words.

We nurses, too, were hesitant about bringing up the possibility of stopping invasive treatments and allowing her to die peacefully.

Anna's father offers another suggestion that we'd all do well to follow. All of us — families and staff — could better communicate our feelings and such things as treatment options and the probabilities of recovery if we got together in a series of conferences led by an ethics committee.

Our hospital has medical-ethics and nursing-ethics committees, but unfortunately they're not utilized as fully as they should be. If we — family, nurses, doctors, social worker — had met regularly with ethics-committee members, I'm sure the haze of misunderstandings would have been cleared. How much anguish this might have spared Anna's family!

Yes, we realize it's too late for them. But, in a different sense, maybe not. We join them in the hope that this is a beginning.

Examining the Ethical Issues

Anna's care raised a number of medical/ethical questions for which there really were no ready answers. The key ones were:

• Was Anna actually in a PVS? Even if not, should she still have been sustained artificially?

- Having seen near-miraculous recoveries, should nurses have offered the family hope when, statistically, the prognosis was very poor?
- Should a nurse try to offer hope when her personal feeling might be that the patient would be "better off" if she'd died?
- Should resources be poured into a case in which there is a very poor prognosis? In England, for instance, where there is socialized medicine, allocating the huge resources needed to sustain Anna's life might not have been permitted.
- How can a nurse help families make a decision — without making it for them?

Additional Readings

Anthony, M. (1986). "No Code: Helping the Family Understand What It Means," *Nursing 86*.16(8):54-55, August.

Beauchamp, T., and Childress, J. (1989). *Principles of Biomedical Ethics*, 3rd edition. New York: Oxford University Press.

Cranford, R. (1984). "Termination of Treatment in the Persistent Vegetative State," *Seminars in Neurology*. 4:1, March.

Dolan, M. (1984). "Where Do You Stand on the Coding Question?" *Nursing 84*. 14(3):42-48, March.

Hastings Center, The. (1988). *Guidelines on the Termination of Life-Sustaining Treatment and the Care of the Dying*. Bloomington, IN: Indiana University Press.

Jimm-Zegeer, L. ((1986). "Brain Edema: Concepts and Nursing Care." In *Acute Neuroscience Nursing: Concepts and Care*, J. Lundgred (ed.). Boston: Jones & Bartlett Publishers, Inc..

Kelly, G. (1958). *Medical-Moral Problems*. St. Louis: Catholic Hospital Association.

Molter, N. (1979). "Needs of Relatives of Critically Ill Patients: A Descriptive Study," *Heart and Lung*. 8(2):332-39, March/April.

Murphy, P. (1986). "When a Non-Death Death Occurs," *Nursing 86*. 16(7):34-39, July.

O'Rourke, K. (ed.). (1986). *Medical Ethics: A Common Ground for Understanding*. St. Louis: Catholic Health Association of the United States.

President's Commission for the Study of Ethical Problems. (1983). *Deciding to Forego Life-Sustaining Treatment*. Washington, DC: U.S. Government Printing Office.

Thompson, J. and Thompson, H. (1985). *Bioethical Decision Making for Nurses*. Norwalk, CT: Appleton & Lange.

U.S. Congress. (1989). *Life-Sustaining Technologies and the Elderly*. OTA-BA-306, Washington, DC: U.S. Government Printing Office.

Veatch, R. (1984). *Death, Dying and the Biological Revolution*. New Haven, CT: Yale University Press.

Wanzer, S., et al. (1984). "The Physician's Responsibility Toward Hopelessly Ill Patients," *New England Journal of Medicine*. 310(15):955-59, April 12.

Health Communication Processes and Theories

Human communication is the primary tool we use to develop a sense of understanding about people and situations. Communication is an adaptive mechanism that helps us survive in a challenging world by enabling us to gather relevant information and elicit cooperation from others. However, it is a deceivingly complex process that occurs every time we respond to a message by assigning meaning to it. We communicate at many different levels, intrapersonally (with ourselves), interpersonally (in dyads), in groups, within organizations, and using a wide range of communication modes and media (speaking face to face with others, writing notes or letters, watching television, using computers to send electronic mail, etc.). We are immersed in a sea of communication (responding to many messages and constantly creating meanings). Since communication is a dynamic ongoing process, we cannot *not* communicate.

Messages derive from many different sources. We send ourselves internal messages both autonomically to regulate our physiological mechanisms and as part of our ongoing intrapersonal dialogue with ourselves (thinking). External messages emanate from our perceptions of our physical environment and our social environment (other people). We use both verbal (the use of words) and nonverbal messages, often together as an inseparable unit. We simultaneously send and receive many messages on many different levels. Every message we send one another has both a content and a relationship dimension. The content dimension of messages refers to the overt subject of a message, while the relationship dimension refers to the inferred implications of messages in defining the nature of our relationships with others. For example, on a relationship level personal communication that shows respect for a person tends to be a humanizing form of interaction, while object communication that shows disrespect toward others tends to be a dehumanizing form of interaction.

Communication is also very fragile. It is easy to misinterpret others, since meanings are in people, not in words, objects or things. It is important to recognize that all people are unique and their individual perceptions of reality and creations of meaning are unique. Communication is also bound to the specific context in which it occurs and is irreversible. Since language is an emergent phenomenon, the denotative (widely accepted) meanings of words change over time, while the connotative (personal) meanings of words differ from person to person. Feedback is often used to help overcome the fragile nature of communication by clarifying communication between people. The readings in this section illustrate the complex and fragile nature of human communication as used in health care. For a broader discussion about the human communication process, please see Kreps and Thornton's *Health Communication: Theory and Practice, Second Edition* (1992).

Lee Ann Glass, a former graduate student at the University of Nevada, Reno, wrote the first reading in this chapter, "Sarah's Story," specifically for this book. This reading dramatically illustrates the importance of human communication in health care. The reading also illustrates the importance of looking at the consumer within a system which is much larger than just the health care arena. The story makes us aware of how content and relationship aspects of messages influence health care interactions. The anger, dissatisfaction, and feeling of powerlessness experienced in this story are vividly presented and remind us of the emotionality of many health care situations.

The second reading is a classic article written by Dean Barnlund, "The Mystification of Meaning: Doctor-Patient Encounters," originally published in the *Journal of Medical Education* in 1976. The article is just as relevant and insightful today as it was when it was first published. Barnlund describes the symbolic aspects of illness as the ways people interpret their health conditions and health care treatments, explaining why physicians and clients are likely to perceive reality very differently. Barnlund argues that effective medical practice must use sensitive and caring communication to treat the symbolic aspects of illness. He explains that traditional medical education has a myopic focus on the physical aspects of illness and is not designed to help physicians meet the communication demands of their jobs. The article concludes with strategies to demystify the symbolic aspects of illness by improving doctor-patient communication. When you read this article, consider implications of the symbolic aspects of illness for the ways you respond to your own health condition. What might you do symbolically to improve the way you typically respond to illness? Since this article was written, many of the issues the author raised have been acknowledged by medical educators and communication scholars. There is, however, much additional research and study needed to enhance the health communication process.

The third reading by Gary Kreps is a paper entitled "Refusing to be a Victim: Rhetorical Strategies for Confronting Cancer," originally presented at a conference on rhetoric and communication at Pennsylvania State University in 1991. This reading builds upon Barnlund's article by challenging people who are living with cancer to symbolically confront their health condition and to use communication as a weapon to fight cancer and enhance their lives. Kreps contends that the ways we use language, especially the use of metaphors, has profound influences on the ways we perceive reality. The reading identifies several communication strategies for coping with cancer at the intrapersonal, interpersonal, group, and organizational levels of human interaction. He also identifies a variety of media and communication technologies that can be used to gather relevant health information. This health communication perspective is not only relevant for confronting cancer but is also relevant for responding to any health challenge.

Kreps, G. L. & Thornton, B. C. (1992). *Health Communication: Theory and Practice* 2nd edition. Prospect Heights, IL: Waveland Press.

3

Sarah's Story

By *Lee Ann Glass*

I don't believe the day will ever come when I don't remember, as vividly as if it were yesterday, the day my daughter was diagnosed with leukemia. It has been four years since that day, and somewhere along the line I've come to accept the fact that this child, who is the greatest joy of my life, has cancer and may possibly die. What I can't accept is what the cost of her health has meant to me and to my family. Through the healing process, I have come to recognize the unresolved anger I have toward members of the health care profession and why that anger is justified. I'm not angry because my daughter has cancer. I'm angry because my daughter's cancer has made us into victims.

When Sarah was ten months old, I took her to our pediatrician for what appeared to be an ear infection. During the course of the appointment, I mentioned that I thought Sarah might be anemic, so a CBC was ordered. After the results of the blood test came back, I was asked to return to the pediatrician's office where I was told that Sarah was anemic, but that our local community didn't have the facilities to diagnose the type of anemia. What I hadn't been told was that leukemia had already been diagnosed. Arrangements were made to send us to a medical center out of state.

Thinking that we were only going to be having some lab work done, we left for Northern California that same day, prepared to spend just a few days. I didn't know that the greatest shock of my life was only a few hours ahead of me, and that my daughter and I would spend nine months in that Northern California city that wasn't our home. When we arrived at the medical center, instead of being sent to the lab as I expected, Sarah was admitted to an isolation room in the Pediatric Intensive Care Unit.

That first evening at the hospital was the beginning of what would be an antagonistic relationship with the hospital staff. After Sarah was admitted and her medical history taken, two arterial lines were started in order that a blood

This article was written especially for this collection. Ms. Glass is in the process of obtaining her social work and law degrees.

exchange could be performed. I voiced my concerns about AIDS to the doctor and also my hesitancy to consent to the procedure because my ex-in-laws are Jehovah's Witnesses. I was immediately threatened that if I didn't consent, the hospital would obtain a court order. I didn't respect my ex-in-laws' chosen religion enough to go to court for it, so I gave my consent. However, the threat had damaged our relationship. After that, there was always the shadow of a thought in my mind that if I didn't do as the doctors ordered, they would take my child from me.

I was given Sarah's diagnosis that evening, but it wasn't until the next day that I met the doctor who would be her primary oncologist. I didn't know at that first meeting that Dr. M. would eventually cause me to really hate someone. I hate her to this day, and if I could bring her to trial for raping my personhood I would. I'm certain that Sarah has survived despite medical treatment by this doctor, not because of it. There was a rumor around the hospital that she used to be a nun. I don't know if that was true, however she certainly had the rigidity and lack of warmth you could picture in a strict "mother superior." I should have ended the relationship the day she walked into my daughter's room and backed away. Sarah had been eating ice cream and reached out to touch Dr. M. I saw my child attempt to establish contact with someone who would have an integral role in her life and be rejected.

One of the first medical terms I learned, after Sarah's diagnosis, was "team approach." The staff at the hospital used that term as if it were their way of giving better care to patients and families. It was a term I soon learned to distrust. As I observed the oncology team, I learned that there wasn't any such thing. There was only Dr. M, head of the department, and her approach. It wasn't hard to see that Dr. M. was the puppeteer and the rest of the staff the puppets. From my own interactions with her, I learned that communication was a facade — no matter what anyone else said, her will would be done.

Sarah's initial hospitalization was seven weeks long. I was told she could not be discharged unless she was able to remain in the area. I was prepared for the possibility that we would have to remain at least six months, so I rented a studio apartment and moved our lives there. As a single parent this was, in many ways, a devastating thing to have to do. I had to leave behind my job, which was our sole source of income. I had to leave my older child behind, in the care of my parents. I had to postpone my plans to return to school. I had no support system, and with an immunosuppressed child I wasn't in any position to go out and develop one. It was worse than being in jail. When Sarah wasn't in the hospital, we were holed up in this tiny apartment with nowhere to go, nothing to do, no one to talk to, and no kind of income that I had any control over. After five months, I couldn't take it anymore. I felt like I was a rubberband that was being pulled tighter and tighter, and I was about to snap. When I told Dr. M. that we had to go home to Nevada I was told that I could leave, but Sarah would have to stay in California in a foster home. I didn't have the strength to fight and I didn't have the strength to leave my child. As it turned out, we stayed another four months. All I can hope is that someday Dr. M. will have to answer to her god for the unwarranted power she exerted on my life, and that she'll be left to rot alone in hell.

The next major incident to occur between a staff member and me amazingly didn't involve Dr. M. This time I was up against Dr. F., who was the co-director of the department. When Sarah was diagnosed, there was an indication that she had central nervous system involvement. One of the ways they treated this involvement was with intrathecal chemotherapy (introducing a chemotherapy drug directly into the spinal fluid). She also had cranial radiation. Since Sarah was so young and such a fighter, she would receive sedation prior to her numerous spinal taps. The problem was that Sarah would react adversely to the sedation. I had heard that another treatment center used general anesthesia when performing spinals on their difficult-to-tap-patients. The next time Sarah was scheduled for a spinal, Dr. F. was the attending physician. I asked him if it would be possible to do Sarah's spinal with general anesthesia. He flatly refused — it was against policy and there was no way they would do it. Well, on this particular occasion Sarah was given a DPT cocktail (a combination of demerol, phenegran and thorazine). This time she went absolutely wild. I thought I was in the examining room with something out of "The Exorcist." She was hissing and scratching, and totally uncontrollable. I was so upset that I was in tears. I asked the doctor if we could wait and do the procedure on another day. He said no, that they were busy and he would go ahead and do it. After several unsuccessful attempts to tap her, instead of giving up, he ordered a megadose of morphine be given. After an hour of waiting the morphine still hadn't calmed her, so we were finally sent home. Later that afternoon I received a telephone call from one of the nurses telling me that Sarah was scheduled in the surgicenter in two days to receive her spinal tap under general anesthesia!

Our return to Nevada brought new problems. Now I was trying to work a full-time job, parent two children and still manage Sarah's medical care on a commuter basis. At first we had to return to California once a month for Sarah's intrathecal chemotherapy. This meant a loss of two days of work and wear and tear on a car that didn't have too many trips left in it. Besides the two days it took us to travel to California and back, I missed quite a bit of time from work as Sarah had low blood counts and was sick frequently. It was quite understandable that my employer was becoming impatient with me since I had just returned from a nine month leave of absence. One of the issues in my next and final battle with Dr. M. revolved around transferring more responsibility for Sarah's care to our local pediatrician, thereby reducing the need for us to commute.

Two other issues were also putting a great deal of stress on my family life. Sarah's protocol called for her to take prednisone, orally, for five days out of each month. A child on prednisone is like a child from hell. They eat incessantly, won't sleep and are unbearably cranky. Not only did my food bill soar astronomically during that week, but it was almost impossible for me to go to work, because if she didn't sleep I sure didn't sleep. I was able to get Dr. M. to schedule Sarah's appointments in California for every other month, but she wouldn't consider taking Sarah off of prednisone. As for the other issue, she evaded and avoided me for six months, until I finally blew.

Sarah had a Broviac catheter, which is a subcutaneous catheter through which blood can be drawn and IV meds administered. The problem with Sarah's Broviac was that I had to do the home nursing care on it. The line had to be flushed twice daily with an anticoagulant and the site had to be cleaned with a sterile technique every other day. I have a very strong-willed child and I was a very stressed mother, so it was almost impossible for me to get the job done. There were times when I couldn't clean the site for days at a time. Sarah would fight because the tape holding the gauze in place would leave her skin raw and irritated. We had tried all sorts of different adhesive products, but nothing worked well. The doctor increased the strength of anticoagulant, so her line would only have to be flushed once a day, but there were times when I couldn't manage that. Nobody wants to be working with a needle around a kicking, fighting child. I'm sure if Sarah had been old enough to communicate and reason, things would have been different.

I asked Dr. M. repeatedly to remove the Broviac, and each time she would placate me by telling me that she would do it at Sarah's next appointment, then Sarah's next appointment would come and it would be the same routine. I asked Sarah's pediatrician to remove it, but he wouldn't because Dr. M. didn't want it done. I called a surgeon and tried to schedule an appointment to have it removed and they refused because we didn't have a referral from our doctor. I was totally helpless. I had consented to have this thing put in my child, yet I couldn't get it taken out. I had reached the point where I was ready to pull it out myself. I felt overwhelmed by trips I couldn't make, prednisone and this damn catheter. Nobody would listen to me. The whole situation culminated in a phone call that left me afraid I was going to have a stroke. My blood pressure had never been that high — I could feel it rising right out of the top of my head. I called Dr. M. to tell her that I wanted the Broviac out, and she started to give me the same old routine. I asked her who would be responsible if the Broviac became infected, and she answered that I would. It wasn't until I screamed that I had asked over and over again to have the Broviac removed as I was unable to care for it properly and that if it did become infected I would sue her for malpractice that she began to listen to me. By then it was too late. I made the decision to transfer Sarah's care to another treatment facility.

Sarah's last appointment at this first hospital was a testimony to her entire treatment at that facility. We left Nevada early in the morning in order to have her in California by 9 a.m. for a clinic appointment and an appointment in the surgicenter. Because she was going to be given general anesthesia, we had to leave Nevada without having breakfast. She had to go to the clinic before the surgicenter, and we were kept waiting there for three hours while Sarah was surrounded by other kids eating food that she couldn't have. The doctors (mighty figures of authority that they are) were standing in the hall arguing over whether or not to admit Sarah because there was pus in her urine. Later it turned out that the results of her tests were wrong. I was totally ignored by Dr. M. when I requested to have Sarah's Broviac removed. We finally made it to the surgicenter, only to find out that the anesthesiologist assigned to us was one I had specifically told Dr. M. and the nurses I would not have work on my child's case. This anesthesiologist is the only one we had had who would not let me stay with Sarah during the procedure for fear I would pass out. I had been going through this for a year, mind you, and hadn't passed out yet. Before I got the chance to protest, Sarah threw up all over the doctor. I could never have expressed my disgust over the entire situation as eloquently. That night we drove on to another northern California city, and the next morning toured what was to become our new treatment center.

I've never had any regrets about changing treatment centers. At the University of California we found the team approach that our former hospital had only claimed existed. Before I made the decision to transfer Sarah's care to UC, I told the staff there that I had three issues that I needed dealt with — 1) the Broviac, 2) prednisone, and 3) the frequency of our trips to California. I was dealt with on all three points. They agreed to take the Broviac out, although once I knew I had the option of having the catheter removed it was no longer a major source of stress, and we managed to keep it in until it became infected two years later, only two weeks shy of Sarah's final treatment. They also agreed to take Sarah off of prednisone if necessary, but the nurse suggested we first try administering the dose once daily, in the evening, rather than twice daily. This approach drastically reduced Sarah's reaction, and we were able to keep her on prednisone until the end of her treatment. Finally, they agreed to Sarah being seen by them every third month, and I knew that was the best we could do. Nothing really changed in Sarah's actual medical care. What changed was that I was no longer locked into a struggle for control. Once I found myself listened to, treated with respect and treated as a competent individual, my attitude changed and Sarah's care definitely improved for the better.

I wish I could say that our story ended here and that the changing of treatment centers brought harmony and balance back into my life, but that's not the case, because what I've told so far is only one aspect of the story. Sarah's illness touched every facet of our lives and sent them spiraling out of control. Of most significance is the way it impacted us economically.

I was divorced before Sarah was born and had been struggling for some time to support two children on one income. We were forced to live with my parents, while I paid off bills that had accrued from my marriage and attempted to save enough money to rent an apartment. When Sarah was diagnosed, I had $500.00 in the bank and a paycheck waiting to be picked up. That isn't a lot of money when your entire life has been reduced to uncertainty. Through the grace of God we've made it, and our needs somehow always seem to be met, but it has been a constant struggle with one bureaucracy or another.

There's a theory in this country that a safety net exists to catch those people who are in need. Most of us are fortunate enough never to have to challenge that theory. There was all sorts of assurance from the hospital social worker, Dr. M. and other hospital staff that programs existed to help us, and I believed them. I didn't know that our country's welfare system is designed to strip its recipients of their pride and devalue them as human beings, through the process of rendering them powerless. All of a sudden, almost every detail of my private life became open to the scrutiny of government agencies. I had to prove myself worthy by filling out reams of paperwork at a time when I was so overcome with grief that I could barely remember my own name, and I had to do this for a sum of money that wasn't enough to live on. I've had to suffer the humiliation of shopping for our groceries with food stamps, knowing that the checker and anyone else watching is probably making a value judgment against this "welfare mother."

I was told by the hospital social worker that I could qualify for Social Security disability benefits for myself on the basis of an emotional disability. Well, grief in its own right doesn't qualify one as emotionally disabled, so in order to prove my worth I had to endure the shame of intense psychological testing. Ironically, I'm unfortunate enough to be sane, thus I suffered that affront to my self-esteem for nothing.

Every time I turn around I have to provide verification of something or other to one agency or another. Because welfare agencies don't know how to communicate with their clients except in a threatening way, these interactions are always unpleasant.

All in all, this has been a terrible experience. Sarah is getting better but our family still suffers from this terrible health care experience. I only hope that people preparing to go into health care, or people already in health care will read this and vow to do better by their patients.

I also wish that more people could realize how a serious illness such as this impacts all aspects of a family's life. Health care is only part of a much larger system that affects all of us. That's why I am going back to school to become a social worker with hopes for a law degree. Maybe I can make someone else's life a little easier when they have a problem like Sarah's.

4

The Mystification of Meaning
Doctor-Patient Encounters
By Dean C. Barnlund

The words "mystique" and "mystify" have a curious affinity in language and life. "Mystique" refers to the magical aura that surrounds objects or persons which endows them with talismanic and magical influence. To "mystify" is to confuse, perplex, or make obscure or difficult to understand. They go together. Mystification is simply the means by which persons are endowed with mystique. While professional mystique seems to be an elusive idea, the process of communication that creates it is subject to systematic analysis.

Examining communicative relationships within the medical profession requires some broad appreciation of the communicative process itself. A good starting point might be this: every person from birth until death is engaged endlessly in a search for meaning. To survive physically and psychically, people must inhabit a world that is fairly stable, relatively free of ambiguity, and reasonably predictable. Though people tolerate occasional doubts, few can accept continuing meaninglessness.

To aid in coping with a chaos of fleeting sensations — what William James called this "blooming, buzzing confusion" — we seek to give events some structure that will render them intelligible. Repeated success in interpreting events contributes to an accumulating set of assumptions on which all future acts depend. These assumptions, as George Kelly once noted, provide templates or guides which every person fits over the realities of life.[1] Gradually people within a culture and within a profession acquire specialized frames of reference which, though they speed the process of judgment, often induce a certain blindness. What is "information" to the specialist may be only "noise" to the lay-person; what the physician regards as "noise," his patient often treats

Reprinted with permission from the Association of American Medical Colleges; *Journal of Medical Education* (now called *Academic Medicine*) 51 (1976): 716-25. At the time of this writing, Dr. Barnlund was a professor in the Department of Speech Communication, School of Humanities, San Francisco State University.

as "information." To the patient excessive thirst may be only an inconvenience, but to the doctor it is a symptom of diabetes; to the examining physician the color of the patient's chart may seem irrelevant, but to the patient it is an ominous sign.

All knowledge of the world is inescapably subjective. In effect, each person stands at the center of his or her own universe of meaning, transforming the flow of sensations into organized and intelligible events. Each of us views the world selectively and fits it to our own past experience and changing purposes. Each notes some details and overlooks others; each finds plausible some relationships and rejects others. Since every interpretation of events rests on fallible senses and personal motives, what is known is always incomplete and always subject to error.

It is tempting in the daily clash of words to forget that it is the perceived world — not the real world — that we talk about, argue about, laugh about, cry about. It is not scalpels and crosses and bedpans that regulate human affairs, but how people construe them that determines what they will think, how they will feel, and what they will do about them. Meanings do not come from the world but are assigned to it by every interpreter, and it is he or she who is the final arbiter of events.

Symbols and Meaning

Language plays a critical role in the construction of the frames of reference through which we view events. It is the most elaborate and most flexible system humans have devised for transforming shapes and sounds into meaningful events. There is wide recognition that the single species-distinguishing attribute of humanity is the capacity to transform experience into symbols. As Langer[2] has emphasized, the brain works as naturally as the kidneys, carrying on a constant process of ideation, even when we are asleep. It follows its own internal law of translating sensory data into symbols to feed our insatiable appetite for meaning.

Life is so permeated with symbolism that it is difficult to imagine any human experience that is not mediated by language. Language tells us what to look for and what to disregard. It suggests causality here and denies it there. It can paralyze us or rouse us to act. It triggers fear and moments later transforms that fear into hope. It is the slender thread by which we overcome our isolation from each other. Yet if words sometimes clarify, they may also distort. If they induce trust, they may also arouse suspicion. If they contribute to insight, they can also lead into error.

Symbolic Dimensions

Symbolic mediation, the intervention of words between people and their experiences, would seem to be an especially sensitive problem in the treatment of human beings. A physical mechanism, a clock or computer, may break down; but any damage to the mechanism is easily identified and repaired without complications. To an animal, injury or disease is simply another physical state. Any suffering is tied directly to disturbances of normal function. Diagnosis has no influence upon the course of the disease, nor does the prognosis complicate recovery.

This is not the case with human beings. Human illness is not only a physical condition but a symbolic one as well. No animal talks itself into becoming sick, suppresses its symptoms because it fears a diagnosis, prolongs recovery because of the symbolic payoff it receives, or spontaneously recovers because it has redefined its situation.

Yet humans do all of these things. They avoid critical examinations that might save their lives. They seek unnecessary treatments and disregard essential ones. They often suffer more from the name of their illness than the physical pain it produces. They suppress some symptoms and invent others. They convert discomfort into excruciating pain and transform extreme suffering into tolerable discomfort. They can go into shock without physical justification and accept a painful death with serenity.

In short, every medical problem is in part a symbolic one. One cannot damage the physical self without injuring the symbolic self, nor can one inflict insult repeatedly on the symbolic self without damaging the physical self. Research on "experimenter influence" and the "placebo effect" convincingly demonstrates that neither physicians nor patients are free of the influence of the way they define their situation. Diagnosis and treatment are in large part symbolic problems, and to ignore this fact may distort or defeat their aims. There is little doubt that how people think about themselves can alter their blood pressure, oxygen needs, and blood chemistry.

The notion that there are a limited number of "psychosomatic" illnesses has gradually given way to the idea that every illness has some psychosomatic reverberations. The broken leg of a young skier may mean a minor inconvenience amply compensated for by increased attention, a flood of sympathetic concern from acquaintances, and special privileges at home and at school. To an older person the same fracture may signal a loss of physical coordination, a sign of aging, or an omen of approaching dependence.

It was once thought that pain was directly proportional to the amount of physical tissue damaged. According to Melzack,[3] this can no longer be assumed, for pain itself depends on the meaning attributed to physical incapacity. This meaning in turn reflects the past experiences and future expectations of the patient. Higher brain functions are capable of modifying or even suppressing signals that accompany physical distress. If every experience of the organism is invested with symbolic significance, it is naive to assume that the most dramatic of life experiences — those involving physical survival itself — are immune to such effects.

To put this another way, for the patient there is no distinction between perceived pain and real pain and between perceived health and real health. This is a dichotomy implied by language but one without counterpart in human experience. It is perceived malfunctions that bring patients to seek care. It is the persistence of such perceptions that keep them in treatment. It is a change in these perceptions that causes them to terminate treatment.

Similarly for the medical profession, it is a perceived disturbance of normal function that mobilizes the physician. He, in turn, acts upon this perception. Through elaborate procedures there is a search to confirm this perception. Investigation may modify or strengthen an initial interpretation. Ultimately it may be shared in part or in full with the patient. Eventually both share a perception of recovery. But all who are involved in the treatment process will base every question, every inference, every recommendation upon meanings assigned to their impressions through the symbols they impose on them. As Friedson has remarked,[4] "illness is a meaning assigned to behavior" and "illness behavior is ordered by that meaning."

One is forced to conclude that there is no patient who does not present the medical profession with, at least in part, a symbolic problem. No illness lacks its semantic dimension. The professional who feels involved exclusively in the maintenance of a physical mechanism and who dismisses the communicative aspect of this work operates on a simplistic and even dangerous premise. Human beings are not merely symbol users; every moment of life is permeated with symbolism.

Obstacles to Communication

The study of communication is concerned with the process by which people attribute meaning to their experience and with their efforts to share such meanings. It focuses upon factors that undermine or facilitate the achievement of common meanings through an exchange of messages. The complexity of medical communication may be intimated by examining some of the more common and more serious barriers to interpersonal understanding in medical settings.

Ego involvement. Less complete communication is likely whenever the topic of conversation is highly ego-involving, such as when one or both parties are fearful of the matter under discussion. Few subjects would appear to arouse as intense feelings as adequacy of the physical or symbolic self. Recent cross-cultural research suggests that the least talked about of all topics are those relating to physical inadequacy, illness, and disease.[5] The anxiety associated with such matters triggers a number of defensive maneuvers, most of which interfere with a clear exchange of meaning. Some people flee and others attack, some refuse to listen and others refuse to talk, some exaggerate and others minimize. But rarely do people comprehend clearly when they are emotionally upset.

Differences in knowledge. Another factor complicating communication resides in the respective power of the communicants. We are beginning to appreciate that information is power. Where knowledge is unequal, where some people have access to the facts and others do not, equality of human relationships is impossible. It is not surprising, therefore, that incomplete and distorted communication surrounds so many encounters between specialists and lay people. To be uninformed is to be communicatively impotent, and this dependent state is not one mature people tolerate gracefully. Rarely is this condition absent between doctors and patients.

Social status. Difficulties are likely, also, when the social distance separating two communicants is great. The greater the disparity in education, income, and social standing, the less people are capable of hearing what was said as it was intended. The presence of higher status figures — parents, teachers, supervisors, police — provokes fear quite apart from whatever they may happen to say. White[6] found his cardiac patients manifesting significantly different levels of tension when he discussed their cases with them in status-aggravating or status-minimizing settings. When status distinctions are emphasized, people avoid contact with each other, withhold information, and distort the meanings intended by the words of others.

Communicative purposes. Status differences are complicated further by differences in point of view arising in part from differences in position and authority. Rarely do communicative purposes overlap completely. Because of distinctive motives, student and teacher do not argue about the "same" grade; nor do husband and wife discuss the "same" child; nor for that matter do physician and patient talk about the "same" X-rays, the "same" disease, the "same" operation, or the "same" fee. Messages acquire much of their meaning from the perspective from which they are uttered. Unless people are sensitive to such differences in purpose or unless these are explicitly discussed, meanings will not coincide since they are anchored in discrepant motives.

Emotional distance. Through conversation people seek some similarity of thought, some congruence of feeling. Words like "rapport," "intimacy," "empathy," and "closeness" are used to describe satisfying encounters with others. But any such meeting of minds is difficult unless both communicants are willing to be "present," not merely available intellectually but totally present as persons. In the interaction of roles, in the encounter of facades, there is no commitment to communication. To give patients the feeling that they are a problem, a disease, or an intriguing curiosity rather than a human being is to undermine the process of sharing meanings. No one has put this point as cogently as Martin Buber.[7] The "I-It" relation, he argues, is demeaning and frustrating for it rests on perceptions of the other as no more than an object. It is only when people confront each other in an "I-Thou" relation that they meet as human beings with respect and mutual concern. When people cultivate emotional distance, they not only prevent any deep sharing of meaning but also arouse animosity and even hatred.

One-way communication. Once communication was regarded as a linear process. Someone, a sender or speaker, transmitted messages to a receiver or listener. Meanings obtained by the receiver were due to the skill of the sender. The sender did the work and the receiver merely paid attention. Any idea could be deposited in the nervous system of another person if one only chose the right words. Now we know better. No one deposits any meaning in the mind of others. Receivers do not passively absorb the intentions of others but creatively interpret what they hear in the light of their own perspectives, their own needs, their own expectations. Reaching any degree of interpersonal understanding requires a process of mutual accommodation. Each person must provide the other with clues to his or her meanings via words and actions. Each must attend to the clues of the other. And each must be prepared to clarify and elaborate his meaning from the viewpoint of the other. This process succeeds to the extent that both parties assume equal responsibility for achieving common meanings.

Yet the prevailing style of interaction from the clinic to the classroom is one-way rather than two-way. And, unfortunately, such channel restrictions impoverish the process and leave receivers confused and impotent. Laboratory studies supply dramatic evidence of the seriousness of this phenomenon where communication flows in only one direction. The simplest instructions are misinterpreted, errors are compounded rather than corrected and morale and human relationships deteriorate. It is easy to appreciate the source of such distortion and friction. Nothing is more demoralizing than to be placed in critical situations and then be prevented from clarifying obscure and confusing messages.

Verbal manipulation. Many efforts to communicate are prompted not by the desire to share or create new meanings but to maneuver the other person into a predetermined decision. Whatever the form of such efforts, from verbal seduction to verbal coercion, they derive from an assumption of moral superiority on the part of one communicant. They also involve disrespect for the integrity of other persons and appropriation of their right to determine their own destiny. Enlarging the communicative responsibility of one person requires some surrender of responsibility by the other. And while such dependency is tolerated by children, adults often find it demeaning and insulting. In a highly manipulative society it is not surprising that most people become adept at recognizing their manipulators. They become suspicious and verbally devious themselves. Thus, communication is often subverted and people antagonized when the authority of their own experience is denied equal weight in the process of making decisions affecting their own survival.

Ambiguity of language. Language itself may introduce barriers to mutual understanding. Through a system of symbols with culturally sanctioned definitions, people seek to share their experience and establish grounds for cooperative action. Yet every communicative code forces the infinity of events into a limited set of categories and fixes appropriate labels to them. "Illness" has perhaps a hundred meanings. "Surgery" may have several dozen. "Fracture" is imprecise. "Cancer" is inexact. If so many words are vague in their reference, messages composed of such ambiguous elements will be even less precise. Nearly every statement can support many legitimate and even contradictory interpretations. In some respects the vocabulary of illness constitutes a special case. Anyone who has attempted to describe a sickness knows the frustration of searching for words to convey the subtle inner disturbances called symptoms. As the great English novelist, Virginia Woolf, once said, "let a sufferer try to describe a pain in his head to a doctor and language at once runs dry." Most people have experienced the communicative paralysis induced by a poverty of words for inner states combined with innocent insistence upon clarity from the doctor.

Language by itself solves nothing. Words can confuse as easily as they clarify. As we have seen, communication is not accomplished by mere listening; it requires a persistent and sensitive effort to solve a mystery whose major clues are provided by words. Common meaning is achieved only through repeated and mutual checking of interpretations. Where people have little appreciation of the ambiguity of words, they remain unaware of the extent to which their remarks can be misunderstood. And they are unlikely to adapt their communicative style to this fact of life.

Role of jargon. Language isolates in another way. Not only do Chinese and Russians speak different languages but also so do males and females, young and old, soldiers and civilians. Every subculture, every trade, and every profession cultivates a dialect of its own. Lawyers, engineers, scientists, accountants and physicians foster their private jargons. These are neither ornament nor luxury; they serve genuine needs; they increase the efficiency of communication within the group; they cultivate rapport among members; they provide a sense of common identity. While contributing to communication within a group, these same dialects when turned outward confuse, frighten, stupefy, alienate. And the more sensitive the topic of conversation, the more such private languages undermine the function for which language was designed. If medical personnel are occasionally puzzled or irritated by the words of economists, lawyers, insurance agents, or musicologists, they might consider the extent to which these same people may be mystified by the diagnostic remarks of physicians.

Pressures of time. Compounding these difficulties is the factor of time. In some ways our humanity seems threatened more by the pace of our lives than by any other single factor. There is no human relationship, no communicative act, that is enriched or improved by speeding it up. It takes time to explain, time to listen, time to dissipate fears, time to assimilate frightening facts, time to prepare for crises, time to enter the experiential world of another person. The urge to hurry must be overcome if people are really serious about preserving the human community.

Significance for Treatment

The factors that complicate the process of sharing meanings are nearly all present in doctor-patient encounters. And most are found here in their most extreme and destructive form. It is here that emotionally disturbing matters, sometimes of life and death, are discussed. It is here that the immense authority and power of one communicant faces the ignorance and impotence of the other. It is here that the need for rapport is largest, yet the emotional distance is likely to be greatest. It is here, too, that critical choice must be made with information which is clothed in an esoteric jargon that obscures and mystifies. And it is here that words are uttered rapidly, even unintelligibly, with little time to clarify or assimilate their meaning. Some of these obstacles to understanding are inherent in illness itself; some derive from the historical roles of physician and patient; others result from the personal communicative style of the physician or are a matter of cultivation by the medical profession.

Yet if people are really serious about improving medical communication, they must resist the appeal of conspiratorial approaches. It is always easier to take sides than to understand — to align ourselves simplistically with child against parent, worker against management, student against teacher, patient against physician. The temptation to search for demons is an addiction the human race has not overcome even in this sophisticated age. The number of villains in the world is probably overestimated, and they are by no means the exclusive property of the medical profession.

Human acts nearly always make sense. They arise from some compromise between private impulse and social expectation. If human behavior is to change, it may be less because we substitute virtue for vice than because we deepen the awareness of people to the total context from which they derive their meanings and motives. The communicative manner of medical specialists may spring less from any malevolent effort to claim omniscience and prestige than from an accident of the role in which medical professionals have cast themselves and been cast by society and from the process by which people are selected and prepared to assume medical responsibilities.

The doctor, as well as the patient, must cope with anxieties surrounding treatment. The doctor may be aware of the seriousness of the case and may know the real limitations of medical knowledge and skill. He may be sensitive to past errors and the possibility of committing further mistakes. There is the danger of making the wrong choice among alternative treatments. There is risk of patient criticism and peer disapproval. If medical personnel sometimes emphasize their authority and status, assert opinions as if they were unassailable, manipulate patients, maintain emotional distance, and discourage patient collaboration, are these not some of the same tactics most people use when threatened and unaware of viable alternatives? Mystification may seem the only constructive way of protecting the patient from undue anxiety in view of the limited assistance that medicine and surgery can provide. It may be used in the hope that mystique can accomplish what science cannot. Mystification permits physicians as well as patients some escape from anxiety, embarrassment, and frustration. This does not justify it, but it may identify its source in the human psyche.

Medical Education

Consider acculturation into the medical profession. How much of this process is designed to promote respect for or insight into human personality? There appears to be minimal effort to assess candidates on their capacity to sustain extensive or intensive human relationships. Yet no profession has daily contact with so wide a spectrum of subcultures, and none exerts influence over such sensitive matters. How many courses are concerned with exploring the ways illness threatens the symbolic as well as physical self? How many class periods focus upon the communicative strategies patients use to cope with imminent threats to their survival? How much time is spent exploring the physician's own communicative style, the assumptions on which it rests, the impulses it reflects, the consequences for those he or she treats?

Throughout training the future physician is preoccupied with the physical properties of the body. Medical training is concerned with anatomy, chemical processes, manifestations of dysfunction, and the consequences of medical and surgical techniques. A vast array of instruments and technologies must be mastered. Is it surprising if later when faced with patients the physician should prefer to deal with their physical rather than psychic symptoms? Will medical specialists not be likely to feel more comfortable and competent handling X-rays, blood samples, printouts, and pathology reports than coping with frightened and distraught personalities? In some offices one gets the impression the physician would prefer never to meet or know the person being treated. If only somehow one could avoid dealing with the human being at all. It is understandable that few patients can effect so neat a surgery between illness and self.

A person's communicative manner derives from his view of human beings. Values are not elusive abstractions; they are manifest in every word. It is difficult to respect the integrity of others and the validity of their experience and at the same time manipulate them — as difficult as it is to see others as mindless children and still collaborate with them as equals. But commitment to humane values is rarely enough, any more than the simple desire to relieve suffering automatically confers diagnostic or surgical talent. Skill must be acquired to translate respect for patients as persons into capacity to engage them communicatively as equals. Communicative skills must be cultivated that respect patients' intelligence, acknowledge their needs, accept their feelings, value their opinions, and promote collaboration in decision making. To achieve this sort of mature relationship demands some recognition of what often occurs under the guise of medical communication and of alternatives for building more effective encounters between physicians and patients.

Research

When one turns to ask what is currently known about communication between medical personnel and patients, the answer is itself mystifying. A phrase will suffice — very little. Here is a profession founded on science, dedicated to truth, committed to inquiry, concerned with the relief of suffering, yet either oblivious to or unwilling to examine its own communicative behavior. Is this simply a mote in an otherwise scientific eye? Or is it a defensive assertion of the medical mystique and the preference to do as one pleases?

If the suffering caused by communicative negligence were a result of some physical disorder, the response would be predictable: organize medical research, underwrite exploratory studies, encourage testing of alternative treatments, and counter the disorder. But when the suffering is a consequence of symbolic disorder — when it arises from the failure to listen, the failure to comprehend, the failure to respect and collaborate — even when such failures result, as they sometimes do, in suffering or death, should there not be an equally vigorous effort to remedy it? It is unfortunate that we have no clear idea of the precise extent of injury to the human personality — or for that matter to the body itself — by the unsought diagnosis, the unasked question, the unreported symptom, the uncomprehended explanation, the disregarded treatment, the incorrectly followed medication. We have only the horror stories so many tell, offset by occasional reports of sensitive and empathic collaboration. While we have some conception of the suffering imposed by broken bones and diseased tissue, we have only the vaguest notion of the damage done through communicative negligence.

This is an area of medicine where the questions far outrun the answers. And the reason there are so few answers is that so few within the field of medicine have raised questions about medical communication. Nearly everyone inside and outside the medical profession affirms that communication with patients deserves study, but few institutions have offered to support such research. To know little about something as complex as interactions between physicians and patients is nothing to apologize for. But to know little and to choose to remain ignorant about it is tragic for the patient and demeaning for the profession.

What are some of the questions that press for answers? We need to know more of the various types of patients and the manner in which they present their condition. There is no reason to assume that high and low income groups, females and males, blacks and whites, educated and uneducated respond in the same way to illness. To claim to respect all patients is nonsense unless medical personnel are willing to meet them on their own communicative terms. There is little reason, also, to assume that all types of illness and injury provoke similar reactions and similar questions or demand similar kinds of involvement. What is a helpful remark in one context may be frightening in another. If patients' reactions bear little resemblance to what seems appropriate, physicians must remember that it is patients' perceptions, not their own, that are the focus of treatment.

We need to know what types of communicative defenses are triggered by illness. It has been suggested that patients tend to be "copers" or "deniers," with the former seeking information in order to assimilate it and the latter avoiding information to keep from being overwhelmed by it. There may be many more ways of handling threatening news than this simple dichotomy suggests. There are, finally, a host of questions concerning the dominant style of the physician. Should it be primarily investigative, informative, supportive, persuasive, collaborative, or therapeutic? At what point and with which patients might each of these contribute to recovery and self-esteem?

Some indication of the kind of investigative work that is possible and its potential is found in a simple exploratory study undertaken in 1970 by Thomas Lonner for a master's thesis at San Francisco State University. It focused on the preoperative and postoperative contacts between one physician and several patients undergoing surgery. The findings are suggestive rather than definitive. But they illustrate the possibilities of such studies.

What the investigator found was this: the physician was genuinely interested in his patients, earnestly tried to provide the care they needed, and attempted to be as clear and informative as possible. His motives were impeccable and his approach was constructive. But it was also clear, in spite of this, that he had only one approach to all patients; that he failed to recognize differences in their reactions to stress; that he was unable to predict their post-operative responses; that he made little effort to confer with them; that he did not adapt verbally, often using words that had no meaning for them; and that when he failed, he sought no explanation for his failure nor did he consider varying his behavior to adapt to this failure. Yet to unsophisticated observers, including some of his patients, he appeared to be an adequate example of the doctor communicating with his patient.

Medical educators, it would appear, must recognize the symbolic and semantic aspects of illness and injury. They must recognize, as well, that all treatment involves a communicative relationship with patients. It is important not only that more intensive efforts be made to investigate this critical relationship between persons seeking treatment and those providing it but also that part of medical training should be developing sensitivity and flexibility in human interaction.

If, as was once written, it is more important to know what manner of man has the disease than to know what disease he has, one might add that to know the manner of man is impossible without appreciating the way he symbolizes his situation. This is a communicative problem of no small dimensions but one for which the medical profession cannot escape some responsibility. It is meanings, not merely physical symptoms, that prompt people to seek or avoid examination, that cause them to withhold or describe their condition, that intensify or minimize their physical discomfort, that prompt them to report or distort reactions to treatment, that lead them to obey or contradict medical advice, that determine ultimately whether they assist or sabotage efforts to cure them. The entire process, from the onset of illness to recovery or death, is invested with symbolism, with meanings that are unique, to every person and to every physical condition. And these meanings, in turn, complicate the conditions that are the focus of treatment. If medical personnel are concerned with the relief of suffering, they can no longer disregard their communicative style with patients. Suffering and the relief of suffering are influenced by symbolic as well as physical acts. Medical personnel are inescapably involved in influencing meanings in some of the most traumatic moments of human existence. Mystification would appear to be a questionable substitute for communicative sensitivity.

Notes

[1] Kelly, G. *The Psychology of Personal Constructs*. New York: Norton, 1955.
[2] Langer, S. *Philosophy in a New Key*. Cambridge, MA: Harvard University Press, 1957.
[3] Melzack, R. The Perception of Pain. *Scientific American* 264 (February 1961):41-49.
[4] Friedson, E. *The Profession of Medicine*. New York: Dodd, Mead, 1972, p. 224.
[5] Barnlund, D. *Public and Private Self in Japan and U.S.* Tokyo: Simul Press, 1975.
[6] White, A. The Patient Sits Down. *Psycoso. Med.* 15 (1953):256-57.
[7] Buber, M. *I and Thou*. New York: Scribner's Sons, 1958.

5

Refusing to be a Victim
Rhetorical Strategies for Confronting Cancer
By Gary L. Kreps

The Cancer-Victim Metaphor

The term "cancer victim" communicates a very unhappy, defeatist metaphor that may be doing a serious disservice to those who are coping with cancer. Victimage conveys helplessness rather than assertiveness, passivity rather than vigor, loss rather than gain; instead, what those who are coping with cancer need most is an active, assertive, fighting attitude toward their health condition (Siegel, 1986). I believe people who are coping with cancer should confront the disease, should be fighters, should take charge, should never give up — should combat cancer (Kreps, 1987).

The metaphor "cancer victim" serves as a negative, self-fulfilling prophesy that undermines the "war against cancer" that I believe should be fought. The metaphor feeds into a pervasive cultural stigma surrounding cancer. This stigma portrays cancer as an evil, relentless juggernaut that kills everything in its path. This does not match the reality of cancer. Cancer is an amorphous term that stands for many different diseases, most of which can be treated effectively (Greenwald and Sondik, 1986). In fact, most people who contract cancer are able to survive the disease and live full and relatively normal lives (General Accounting Office, 1987).

Every health care problem has both a physical and a symbolic dimension (Barnlund, 1976). The physical and the symbolic are interdependent; they influence one another. The way people symbolically interpret their health conditions has a direct influence on their actual physical conditions (Cousins, 1979; Frank, 1975). If consumers believe cancer will kill them, they increase

This article was orginally presented at The Pennsylvania State University Conference on Rhetoric and Composition, State College, PA, July 10-13, 1991. Dr. Kreps teaches in the fields of organizational and health communication at Northern Illinois University.

the chances it probably will. If they believe they can overcome cancer, they increase the chances they probably can. The metaphors people use to describe themselves encourage them to take a constructive or destructive attitude towards their lives, becoming therapeutic or nontherapeutic self-fulfilling prophesies (Norton, 1989, 1986). Perhaps some more constructive metaphors to use to describe an active perspective for coping with cancer might be "struggling" or "fighting cancer," or even "beating" or "overcoming cancer."

The terms people use to define themselves directly influence the way they feel about themselves and the behaviors in which they engage. The "cancer victim" self-definition limits consumers' potential to cope effectively with cancer by minimizing their perceptions of personal control over their lives. The victim metaphor minimizes personal control and encourages fatalistic resignation to the all-powerful, controlling influences of eternal forces. Brenders (1987) suggests that "perceptions of control help the person to act in proactive, goal-directed ways, as opposed to reactive self-limiting, and goal-destructive ways" (p. 90). In this paper, I will describe rhetorical strategies which people can use to increase their control over cancer.

The Strategic Role of Communication in Fighting Cancer

Communication is a primary tool for people who are overcoming cancer to use in accomplishing their health promoting goals. Communication enables them to gather relevant information to guide their health maintaining strategies, as well as to elicit cooperation from others in fighting cancer (Kreps, 1988b). Information is powerful! Accurate and timely information can liberate health care consumers by helping them make enlightened choices, while insufficient levels of information limit the choices and options available to them. I advocate the strategic use of communication for seeking and sharing relevant information in combatting cancer (Kreps, 1987).

There are two primary kinds of information needed to combat cancer — "content"-oriented information about cancer and "relationship"-oriented information about the emotional aspects of health and illness (Kreps & Thornton, 1984). Content and relationship information are important elements in therapeutic communication that enable people to understand and overcome their problems. Content information can provide cancer-fighters with relevant data concerning the current state of knowledge available about their specific disease and the most effective treatment strategies available to them. Relationship information can provide cancer-fighters with emotional support and encouragement to help them combat cancer.

Health Care Providers as Information Sources

Potentially rich sources of content and relationship information for cancer-fighters are their health care providers and other health care system representatives. Yet, the health care system is not often very "user-friendly" and is not geared to provide consumers with all of the information they need for effectively combatting cancer (Waitzkin and Stoekle, 1972; 1976). Even the term "patient," commonly used in most health care systems, may limit the information available to cancer-fighters. Just like the limiting metaphor of "cancer victim," the term "patient" conveys a passive, docile perspective to health care. "Do with me what you will. I entrust my life to you." Patients don't rock the boat; they don't seek information; they don't make active decisions; they are patient and have blind faith in their health care providers.

I reject this passive perspective on health care and advocate an active fighting perspective. Health care consumers have legal and moral rights to relevant health information. Health care providers are required to ensure their clients have "informed consent" (ability to make knowledgeable choices about the health care services they wish to receive) before choosing health care treatments. Yet, cancer patients are too often pressured by their physicians into agreeing immediately to follow specific treatment regimens without receiving full information about alternative treatment choices or about the long-term physical and psychological implications of the treatments advocated (Greenfield, Kaplan, and Ware, 1985; Waitzkin and Stoekle, 1972; 1976).

The research literature identifies many barriers to effective communication of health information between doctors and clients (Kreps, 1988a; Speedling and Rose, 1985). Typically, physicians are not well trained in the intricacies of communicating relevant information to consumers or in eliciting full disclosure of information from their clients (Barnlund, 1976; Kreps, 1988a; 1988b). Medical training focuses far more on understanding medical information than on the ability to convey or to seek information from consumers. Due to limited training in health communication skills, even physicians who want to disclose relevant health information to their clients are not effective at doing so. Compounding this problem is the fact that consumers often feel uncomfortable and intimidated about seeking information from their physicians. Even when consumers do not understand their physicians, they are often too embarrassed to ask for clarification. Consumers may also withhold relevant information about their health conditions from their doctors because they feel the information is irrelevant, embarrassing, or they don't have the opportunity or abilities to convey the information.

Cancer-fighters need relevant health information. To get information from physicians, I encourage cancer-fighters to establish meaningful personal relationships with their physicians. They should get to know their doctors and help their doctors get to know them. They should reach a first name basis with their doctors, eliminating as much emotional, educational, and status distance between doctors and clients as possible. Consumers should let their doctors know they are fighters and want information. This will help consumers acquire both content-and relationship-oriented information from their physicians. Consumers should become actively involved in monitoring their treatment and making treatment choices. They should seek the latest information about cancer treatment research. If they find that their physicians will not or cannot give them the information they need, they should seek information from other sources. They should seek second opinions. Perhaps consumers should fire doctors that do not provide them with the health information they need and hire other doctors who will share relevant information. Consumers should be in charge of their own treatment.

Formal and Informal Sources of Health Information

In addition to physicians, there are many good formal and informal sources of health information available. Cancer fighters should actively seek relevant information from all available sources. They should get to know the different members of their health care teams (nurses, therapists, social workers, pharmacists, etc.). They should enlist help from health team members, family members, or friends to act as advocates in acquiring relevant information and in getting their needs communicated within the health care system. It is difficult for a consumer to be powerful when incarcerated in a hospital bed wearing IV tubes and a hospital gown. Advocates become consumers' personal representatives within the health care system.

Family members should be encouraged to provide support and encouragement to relatives in their fight against cancer. The family can be an important source of relationship information in combatting cancer (Wortman and Dunkel-Schetter, 1979). Similarly, friends and co-workers can provide emotional support and encouragement (Kreps, 1988c). Family members, friends, and co-workers can help make cancer-fighters' lives as full and satisfying as possible, giving them the strength to wage war with cancer (Sullivan and Reardon, 1986).

There are also many institutional sources of information available to cancer-fighters. The National Cancer Institute's Cancer Information Service (CIS) has a toll-free cancer information hotline (1-800-For-Cancer) to provide the public with the latest content information about cancer treatment. The CIS hotline has access to the Physician Data Query (PDQ) cancer treatment information database that contains state-of-the-art information about cancer treatment and can provide information from PDQ to callers. PDQ can also be accessed from most medical and hospital libraries that subscribe to the MEDLARS database system of the National Library of Medicine. The American Cancer Society also has a toll-free answer line (1-800-ACS-2345) that provides callers with cancer information and referral for support services. Specialized peer-support groups like Make Today Count, Exceptional Cancer Patients, and the National Coalition for Cancer Survivorship are available to provide cancer-fighters with relevant content and relationship information.

Conclusion

In summary, I advocate that consumers take personal charge of their own health care by using communication to seek and send relevant information. The most therapeutic method for coping with cancer is to fight it (Kreps, 1987). Health information can help consumers fight cancer by helping them make the best possible choices in cancer care. Communication should be used to gather information, enlist support, and elicit cooperation from others in resisting and overcoming cancer and making the health care system work for consumers rather than against them.

References

Barnlund, D. (1976). The mystification of meaning: doctor-patient encounters. *Journal of Medical Education* 51, 716-25.

Brenders, D. (1987). Perceived control: Foundations and directions for communication research. In M. McLaughlin (ed.). *Communication Yearbook* 10, (pp.86-116). Newbury Park, CA.

Cousins, N. (1979). *Anatomy of an illness as perceived by the patient.* New York: W. W. Norton.

Frank, J. (1975). The faith that heals. *Johns Hopkins Medical Journal* 137, 127-31.

General Accounting Office. (1987). *Cancer patient survival: What progress has been made.* Washington, DC: GAO, Publication No. GAO/PEMD-8713.

Greenfield, P., Kaplan, S., and Ware, J. (1985). Expanding patient involvement in care: Effects on patient outcomes. *Annals of Internal Medicine* 102, 520-28.

Greenwald, P. and Sondik, E. (eds.). (1986). *Cancer control objectives for the nation: 1985-2000.* Bethesda, MD: National Cancer Institute, NCI Monographs No. 2.

Kreps, G. (1987). Communication, cancer, and the therapeutic process. In L. Robbins, B.M. Goff, and L. Miller (eds.). *Cancer and the workplace: Strategies for support and survival,* (pp. 15-19). New Brunswick, NJ: Rutgers University.

Kreps, G. (1988a). Relational communication in health care. *Southern Speech Communication Journal* 53, 344-59.

Kreps, G. (1988b). The pervasive role of information in health and health care: Implications for health communication policy. In J. Anderson (ed.), *Communication Yearbook* 11, (238-76). Newbury Park, CA: Sage.

Kreps, G. (1988c). Communicating about death. *Journal of Communication Therapy* 4, 2-13.

Kreps, G. and Thornton, B. (1984). *Health Communication.* New York: Longman.

Norton, C.S. (1989). *Life metaphors.* Carbondale, IL: Southern Illinois University Press.

Norton, C.S. (1986). The therapeutic functions of metaphor. *Journal of Communication Therapy* 3, 138-63.

Siegel, B. (1986). Love, medicine, and miracles. New York: Harper and Row.

Speedling, E. and Rose, D. (1985). Building an effective doctor-patient relationship: From patient satisfaction to patient participation. *Social Science and Medicine* 21, 115-20.

Sullivan, C. and Reardon, K. (1986). Social support satisfaction and health locus of control: Discriminators of breast cancer patients' styles of coping. In M. McLaughlin (ed.), *Communication Yearbook* 9, (pp. 707-22). Beverly Hills, CA: Sage.

Waitzkin, H. and Stoekle, J. (1972). The communication of information about illness. *Advances in Psychosomatic Medicine* 8, 180-215.

Waitzkin, H. and Stoekle, J. (1976). Information control and the micropolitics of health care: Summary of an ongoing research project. *Social Science and Medicine* 10, 263-76.

Wortman, C. and Dunkel-Schetter, C. (1979). Interpersonal relationships and cancer. *Journal of Social Issues* 35, 132-55.

CHAPTER
3

The Interpersonal Health Communication Context

Interpersonal communication performs many important functions in health care. It is at the interpersonal level of communication that health care interviews are conducted. (Health care interviews are the primary formal context for information exchange between health care providers and consumers.) Interpersonal communication is also used to establish effective working relationships between interdependent health care providers, as well as between consumers and providers. Relationship development is important in health care because effective relationships enhance trust, disclosure, and cooperation between relational partners.

To develop effective relationships implicit contracts (unwritten and often unspoken agreements) are established and updated to guide the mutual fulfillment of relational expectations between interpersonal communicators. For example, implicit contracts guide the kinds of language that relational partners use with one another, the level of intimacy they express, the conversational topics that are discussed, even the ways they touch one another. If these implicit contracts (agreements) are not recognized and followed the communicators will become frustrated and dissatisfied with interacting with each other. However, the more implicit contracts are followed the more comfortable and satisfied communicators feel with one another.

In effective relationships interpersonal communication is often used to communicate therapeutically. Therapeutic communication provides relational partners with personal insight and reorientation and empowers them to solve problems and make decisions about their lives (Barnlund, 1968; Kreps & Thornton, 1992). Therapeutic communicators provide their relational partners with social support and help them cope with difficult situations. It is important for health care providers to communicate therapeutically with their clients, as well as with their co-workers. Therapeutic communication is also expressed informally within families and between friends in everyday life as an important way of helping and comforting relational partners. This section of the book describes the importance of relational interaction in health care and describes how effective interpersonal communication can be used to enhance health care delivery.

The first reading in this chapter, "Relational Communication in Health Care" written by Gary Kreps, was published originally as an article in the *Southern Communication Journal*. It examines current knowledge about the role of interpersonal communication in the development and maintenance of relationships and describes applications of such knowledge for health care relationships.

The second reading, "Health Care Providers and Consumers: Making Decisions Together," written by Deborah Ballard-Reisch specifically for this book, examines the communication rights and responsibilities that providers and consumers bring to health care interactions. Ballard-Reisch presents an insightful model of participative decision making in doctor-client interactions that describes the interaction as a relational negotiation. As you review this reading, think about how you typically communicate in doctor-client interactions. Which negotiation styles are you most likely to utilize? The reading contends that participative decision making between doctors and clients can lead to therapeutic outcomes. How do you think participative decision making can be encouraged?

Barnlund, D. (1968). Therapeutic communication. In D. Barnlund (ed.), *Interpersonal Communication* (pp. 613-645). Boston: Houghton-Mifflin.

Kreps, G. L. & Thornton, B. C. (1992). *Health Communication: Theory and Practice* 2nd edition. Prospect Heights, IL: Waveland Press.

6

Relational Communication in Health Care

By Gary L. Kreps

Research has demonstrated that interpersonal communication between health care providers and consumers clearly plays an important role in health care delivery (Arntson, 1985; Greenfield, Kaplan & Ware, 1985; Thompson, 1984; Waitzkin, 1984). Effective communication can promote the delivery of high quality health care, while ineffective communication can seriously deter the quality of health care delivery (Cline, 1983; Kreps & Thornton, 1984). It is at the interpersonal level of health communication that meaningful relationships are established between those individuals who are seeking and those who are providing health care services. Relationship development in health care facilitates exchange of relevant health information, coordination of efforts, and provision of emotional support between interdependent health care consumers and providers (Kreps, 1988). Ineffective interpersonal communication has been shown to lead to dissatisfaction with health care services (Korsch & Negrete, 1972), alienation between health care providers and consumers (Lane, 1981), and excessive competition between health care providers (Frank, 1961; Friedson, 1970). This article provides a review and analysis of major topics of health communication research related to relational communication, ultimately suggesting an integrating perspective for applying health communication knowledge to enhancing the quality of health communication practice.

Relating Relational Communication to Health Communication

Relational communication is a well developed area of communication inquiry, with many studies conducted and theoretical models developed concerning

Reprinted by permission of the Southern States Communication Association from the *Southern Communication Journal 53*: 344-359, 1988.

the role human communication performs in establishing and maintaining human relationships. Relational communication research and theory has focused on the following six general topics and issues:

1. the initiation and development of relationships (Altman & Taylor, 1973; Berger & Calabrese, 1975; Berger, Gardner, Clatterbuck & Schulman, 1976; Duck, 1976; Fisher & Drecksel, 1983; Millar & Rogers, 1976; Parks, 1977; Parks & Adelman, 1983);

2. the maintenance and repair of relationships (Baxter & Dindia, 1987; Fitzpatrick & Best, 1979; Krayer & O'Hair, 1987; O'Hair & Krayer, 1987);

3. the deterioration and dissolution of relationships (Baxter, 1979, 1982; Cody, 1982; Dindia & Baxter, 1987; Duck, 1982);

4. strategies for analyzing relational communication (Courtwright, Millar & Rogers-Millar, 1979; Folger & Poole, 1982; Rogers & Farace, 1975);

5. relational competence (Cupach & Spitzberg, 1981; Spitzberg, 1984; Spitzberg & Hecht, 1984);

6. self-disclosure in relationships (Baxter, 1979; Wheeless, 1976, 1977; Wheeless & Gratz, 1976).

Few communication researchers have applied relational communication theory to dyadic behavior in health care, although the development of effective provider-consumer relationships is a central concern in health care delivery (O'Hair, O'Hair, & Kontas, 1985). Several topics of health communication research are concerned with the role of interpersonal communication in health care relationships and are ripe for relational communication analysis. Many health communication studies have examined specific interpersonal communication practices and problems related to relational communication. The study of therapeutic communication has largely been concerned with identifying the specific dyadic communication characteristics leading to therapeutic outcomes. The early work of Ruesch (1957, 1961, 1963), Ruesch and Bateson (1951), Rogers (1951, 1957, 1967), and Carkhuff (1967) described the communication characteristics of helpers that lead to therapeutic outcomes. More recently, studies by Pettegrew (1977), Pettegrew and Thomas (1978), Burleson (1983), Northouse (1977), and Rossiter (1975), explored specific strategies used in effective therapeutic communication such as communicating empathetically and comfortingly with others. The approaches taken and conclusions reached by these studies of therapeutic communication have been diverse, yet all studies support the contention that establishing and maintaining supportive and caring communication relationships increases therapeutic outcomes for communicators.

A great deal of study has centered around planning and directing relationship development in provider-patient interviews (Arntson, Droge, & Fassl, 1978; Carroll & Monroe, 1980; Cassata, Conroe & Clements, 1977; Foley & Sharf,

1981; Hawes, 1972a, 1972b; Hawes & Foley, 1973). Much of this research has examined interpersonal communication patterns in interviews, identified specific communication characteristics used by health care providers to control interview communication, and developed strategies to help health care providers establish rapport and elicit full and accurate information from health care consumers. The research concerning health care interviews has tended to be pragmatic and applied to realistic concerns of information exchange in interview situations. Its applicability to a wider range of relational health communication contexts other than provider/consumer interviews, however, such as interprofessional health care relationships and peer support relationships, has been limited.

A large body of health communication research has addressed specific recurring problems in health care by linking these problems to interpersonal communication inadequacies. For example, five different topic areas of such research include:

1. low levels of patient compliance have been linked to the failure to establish effective provider/patient communication relationships (Charney, 1972; DiMatteo, 1979; Lane, 1983, 1982; Stone, 1979);

2. miscommunication and misinformation in health care have been related to inaccurate interpersonal interpretations, ineffective and manipulative message strategies and failures to seek and utilize interpersonal feedback between health communicators (Golden & Johnson, 1970; Ley, 1972);

3. insensitivity in health care has been related to low levels of interpersonal respect, attempts for relational control, and inability to accurately interpret nonverbal messages (Daly & Hulka, 1975 ; Kane & Deuschle, 1967; Korsch, Gozzi & Francis, 1968; Korsch & Negrete, 1972; Lane, 1982);

4. unrealistic and unfulfilled patient expectations have been linked to cultural stereotypes, misinterpretations of relational needs, and inflexible relational role performances (Blackwell, 1967; Fuller & Quesada, 1973; Mechanic, 1972; Myerhoff & Larson, 1965; Walker, 1973);

5. dissatisfaction with health care by both providers and consumers have been tied to failures to express interpersonal empathy and to issues of relational dominance and dehumanization (Ben-Sira, 1976; Kane & Deuschle, 1967; Korsch, Gozzi & Francis, 1968; Korsch & Negrete, 1972; Lane, 1983; Street & Wiemann, 1987).

These five problem-oriented topic areas of health communication research highlight the important role of human communication in establishing and maintaining effective health care relationships, suggesting that the effectiveness of communication relationships directly influences the success of health care (Greenfield, Kaplan & Ware, 1985; Kreps, 1988; Street & Wiemann, 1987). The studies reviewed identify several glaring deficiencies in interpersonal communication in health care relationships. Regrettably, however, most of these studies have not gone beyond merely identifying communication problem areas. The next step is to apply this research to planning, developing, and implementing strategies for improving interpersonal health communication and relieving these relational deficiencies.

An intriguing new area of health communication research has examined the social support functions of interpersonal communication in health care (Albrecht & Adelman, 1984; Dickson-Markman & Shern, 1984; Droge, Arntson & Norton, 1981; Gottlieb, 1981; Query, 1987). These studies have demonstrated the need for expressive social communication contacts with others to help maintain individual well-being and psychological health. The social support construct has become very important as the American public has gradually taken increasingly more responsibility for its own health and health care, depended more on peers for health information, and begun widespread use of self-help groups for emotional, psychological, and informational health care services (Kreps, 1988). Unfortunately, social support research remains a largely unintegrated and unrefined area of inquiry with few consistent findings; because diverse methods of operationalization have been used, comparisons of findings have been limited and this potentially rich area of study remains relatively underdeveloped (Query, 1987).

Limitations of Past Research

Relational aspects of health communication is a relatively recent area of research. Many key issues have not been fully explored, while other topics, such as compliance, have received the lion's share of research attention. Much of the research that has been conducted on relational issues in health communication has not been well integrated. Research has tended to focus on several small parts of the interpersonal health communication process without linking these parts together into meaningful configurations. Work needs to be done to examine, explain, and integrate past health communication research (Arntson, 1985; Thompson, 1984).

The focus of attention in past health communication research has overwhelmingly been on the interpersonal communication needs of health care providers, often ignoring the interpersonal communication needs of health care consumers (Thompson, 1984). (A notable exception to this trend has been the recent research concerning social support networks that primarily examines the communication needs of health care consumers acting as providers.) Just as many applied organizational communication studies have tended to adopt a management orientation in terms of the researchers they serve with their research (Pacanowsky & O'Donnell-Trujillo, 1982), health communication research has often adopted a health care provider orientation. For example, compliance research has focused on how providers can get consumers to follow instructions. The term "compliance" itself suggests a one-way power orientation with the consumer being responsible to the provider. Kreps and Thornton (1984) suggest redefining the issue of compliance into a relational issue of "cooperation" to fully take into account the interdependent communicative functioning of health care provider and consumer. Clearly, consumers as well as providers of health care have important and challenging interpersonal communication needs in health care. Health care consumers need to use interpersonal communication skills to:

1. gather relevant health information about their health problems and treatments;

2. elicit cooperation and respect from the health care providers that serve them;

3. collaborate with others to make complex and far-reaching health care decisions;

4. influence others to cope with the often-restrictive bureaucracy of the health care system;

5. cope symbolically with their health problems.

To help consumers achieve these interpersonal goals, health communication research should focus on how to increase the effectiveness of both consumers' and providers' communication in health care relationships.

In addition to the marked overemphasis on studying health care providers at the expense of health care consumers, past studies in health communication have not fully examined the different communication needs and problems of different specialized areas of health care delivery. Past research has primarily been designed to examine the role of interpersonal communication in the two health professional fields of medicine and nursing, neglecting such specialized health service areas as dentistry, physical and occupational therapy, social work, pharmacy, health care administration, and other allied health fields (Thompson, 1984). Certainly human communication is an influential process in these other areas of health care service. Interprofessional communication between the many different specialized health care fields is also an important, yet largely neglected, topic of study (Frank, 1961; Friedson, 1970; Kreps and Thornton, 1984).

Past health communication research has tended to neglect several important populations of health care consumers, including the aged (Kreps, 1986). The aged are by far the largest group of health care consumers in the United States (Pegels, 1980). As people grow old, their physical condition weakens and they are generally more prone to experience health care problems than their younger counterparts (Weg, 1975). Moreover, the health care problems the elderly face are often chronic and debilitating, necessitating long-term health care treatment, often to the point of institutionalization within health care and quasi-health care service organizations like hospitals, sanitariums, convalescent centers, or nursing homes. The aged suffer from serious interpersonal health communication problems due to issues of stigmatization, paternalism, alienation, boredom, and fraud (Kreps, 1986). Future research should be designed to examine the health communication needs of the aged.

As mentioned earlier, past research has focused more often on description of interpersonal health communication patterns, issues, and problems, than on examining specific directions for improving relational health communication. Due to the youth of health communication inquiry, a descriptive research approach may be necessary to clearly define the issues under investigation. Certainly health care consumers would want and expect their health care providers to carefully diagnose health problems before prescribing health care remedies. Applied communication research should work in a similar fashion by describing the nature of health communication issues before prescribing strategies for improvement. In doing a good job of description, we can be confident that the improvement strategies we design are appropriate to the specific problems that limit the effectiveness of relational health communication. The agenda for future inquiry on health communication should address our current state of disciplinary development and description of relational health communication. Work needs to be done to identify what it is we presently know about relational communication in health care, categorizing and integrating research findings, and initiating a move in health communication research from an emphasis on description to emphases on integration, elaboration, application and development. A fruitful area for such integration and development is in the identification and implementation of interpersonal communication competencies for health care providers and consumers.

Health Communication Competencies: A Research Agenda

Both health care providers and consumers depend on their communication to gather information in health care situations (Maibach & Kreps, 1986). However, the role of communication and information in health care is so ubiquitous, equivocal, and pervasive that it is often taken for granted, and complexities and subtleties of health communication are often unnoticed, incompletely analyzed, and ineffectively used (Kreps, 1988). Communication competency, the ability to effectively utilize interpersonal relations skills to seek and share relevant health information, is as important for health care providers and consumers as technical competence (Kreps, 1988; Maibach & Kreps, 1986; Ruben, 1976; Ruben & Bowman, 1986).

Past research supports the need for health communication competencies. Results of research on relational aspects of health care (discussed earlier) clearly demonstrate that the effectiveness of interpersonal communication relationships established between health care providers and consumers have a major influence on the level of success of health care treatment. The provider-client relationship exerts a strong influence on the outcomes and satisfaction people derive from health care experiences. Human communication processes enable health care consumers and providers to gather and interpret pertinent information for accomplishing health care delivery objectives. Competent communication encourages cooperation between health care providers and consumers, and facilitates the sharing of relevant information necessary to accomplish health evaluation and maintenance (Babbie, 1973; Kreps, 1988).

A considerable body of literature has addressed the issue of communication competence, especially examining the nature of communication competence and the manner in which communication competencies are developed in different social contexts (Bochner & Kelly, 1974; Bostrom, 1984; Spitzberg & Cupach, 1984; Wiemann, 1977). This research indicates that communication competence is a multidimensional construct based on a wide range of communication abilities that are developed from a combination of communication knowledge and skills. Moreover, communication competence is situationally-bound and depends on the abilities of communicators to adapt to one another in specific relational settings (Ruben, 1976).

Several studies have attempted to identify various dimensions of communication competence that are important in specific contexts, such as the ability to communicate with empathy (Carkhuff, 1969; Fine & Therrien, 1977; Rogers, 1951), use nonjudgmental listening (Cline, 1983; Gibb, 1961; Ruben & Kealy, 1979), demonstrate interpersonal respect (Rogers, 1951; Ruben & Kealy, 1979), display informational congruence between message intended and message received (Powers & Lowry, 1984), and manage interactions (Ruben & Kealy, 1979; Wiemann, 1977). By integrating research findings from communication competence research with data concerning relational aspects of health communication, interpersonal health communication competencies can be identified.

The results of much of the past health communication and relational communication research and theory reviewed in this article can be summarized in an initial model of relational health communication competence built upon an existing model of the interdependence of health communicators developed by Kreps and Thornton (1984, p. 4). The Kreps and Thornton model of the "Health Care Delivery System Wheel" (see Figure 1) is a representation of a wagon wheel with many different spokes. The spokes of the wheel represent interdependent health care providers, while the hub of the wheel represents the health care consumer, demonstrating that the health care system revolves around the consumer. The model illustrates the interdependent communication relationships that exist between providers and consumers in the delivery of health care. Communication must flow between the different spokes (providers) of the wheel and between the spokes and the hub (consumers) of the wheel for effective health care delivery. By adding to this model the relational communication competencies of health care providers and consumers, we can begin to see how the wheel is powered to accomplish health care delivery goals.

Figure 1

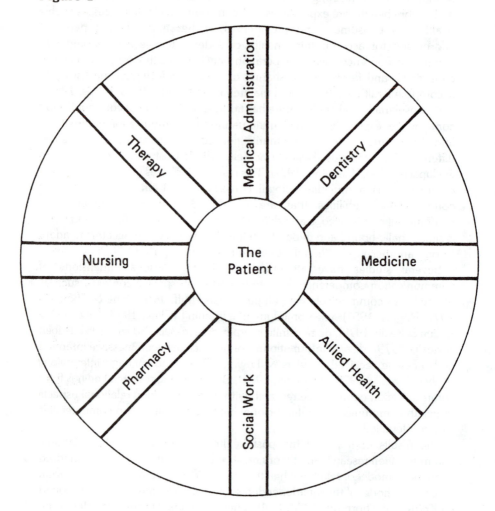

The Health-Care Delivery System Wheel

In the model of Relational Health Communication Competence (see Figure 2) the hub representing the consumer and the spokes representing the providers are widened to account for the level of relational communication competence engendered by the individuals performing these interdependent health care roles. Relational health communication competence embodies specific provider and consumer communication knowledge and skills, such as empathy, nonjudgmental listening, respect, message congruence and interaction management. The terrain upon which the wheel rolls is representative of the

Figure 2

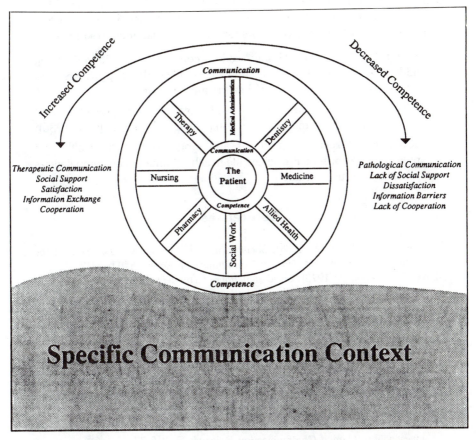

Model of Relational Health Communication Competence

specific health care context within which providers and consumers interact. Certain contexts may be steeper and more difficult to traverse than other contexts. These contexts will demand high levels of relational communication competence between providers and consumers to enable the wheel to roll forward to accomplish health communication goals, such as increased interpersonal satisfaction, therapeutic communication outcomes, cooperation between providers and consumers, social support and effective information exchange. Insufficient levels of communication competence will cause the wheel to stand still or worse, roll backwards, failing to fulfill health communication goals.

Promoting health care provider and consumer communication competencies can help improve the quality of health care and can increase the satisfaction consumers and providers derive from health care situations. This major implication of the Relational Health Communication Competence Model is clearly supported by health communication research and theory (Cline, 1983; Cline & Cardosi, 1983; Kreps & Thornton, 1984; Morse & Piland, 1981; Worobey & Cummings, 1984). Future research can build upon this model by:

1. testing the suggested communication competencies and identifying additional communication competencies needed by providers and consumers in a wide range of health care contexts;

2. establishing clear performance-based measures for providers' and consumers' health communication competencies (Kreps & Query, 1986);

3. developing educational strategies and programs to help health care providers and consumers cultivate the health communication competencies identified through research.

References

Albrecht, T. & Adelman, M. (1984). Social support and life stress: New directions for communication research. *Human Communication Research*, 11, 3-32.

Altman, I. & Taylor, D. (1973). *Social penetration: The development of interpersonal relationships*. New York: Holt, Rinehart, and Winston.

Arntson, P. (1985). Future research in health communication. *Journal of Applied Communication Research*, 13, 118-30.

Arntson, P., Droge, D. & Fassl, H. (1978). Pediatrician-parent communication: Final report. In B. Ruben (ed.), *Communication yearbook 2*, (pp. 505-22). New Brunswick, NJ: Transaction.

Babbie, S. (1973). *Medical communication requirements*. Springfield, VA: US Pacific.

Baxter, L. (1982). Strategies for ending relationships: Two studies. *Western Journal of Speech Communication*, 46, 223-41.

Baxter, L. (1979). Self disclosure as relational disengagement strategy: An exploratory investigation. *Human Communication Research*, 5, 215-22.

Baxter, L. & Dindia, K. (1987, May). *Marital partners' perceptions of marital maintenance and repair strategies*. Paper presented at the International Communication Association convention, Montreal.

Ben-Sira, Z. (1976). The function of the professional's affective behavior in client satisfaction: A revised approach to social interaction theory. *Journal of Health and Social Behavior*, 17, 3-11.

Berger, C. & Calabrese, R. (1975). Some explorations in initial interaction and beyond: Toward a developmental theory of interpersonal communication. *Human Communication Research*, 1, 99-112.

Berger, C., Gardner, R., Clatterbuck, G. & Schulman, L. (1976). Perceptions of information sequencing in relationship development. *Human Communication Research*, 3, 29-46.

Blackwell, B. (1967). Upper middle class adult expectations about entering the sick role for physical and psychiatric dysfunctions. *Journal of Health and Social Behavior*, 8, 83-95.

Bochner, A., & Kelly, C. (1974). Interpersonal competence: Rationale, philosophy, and implementation of a conceptual framework. *Speech Teacher*, 23, 279-301.

Bostrom, R. (ed). (1984). *Competence in communication*. Beverly Hills, CA: Sage.

Burleson, B. (1983). Social cognition, empathic motivation, and adults' comforting strategies. *Human Communication Research*, 10, 295-304.

Carkhuff, R. (1969). *Helping and human relations*, Vol. 1. New York: Holt, Rinehart & Winston.

Carkhuff, R. (1967). Toward a comprehensive model of facilitative interpersonal processes. *Journal of Counseling Psychology*, 14, 67-72.

Carroll, J. & Monroe, J. (1980). Teaching clinical interviewing in the health professions: A review of empirical research. *Evaluation and the Health Professions*, 3, 21-45.

Cassata, D., Conroe, R. & Clements, P. (1977). A program for enhancing medical interviewing using videotape feedback in the family practice residency. *Journal of Family Practice*, 4, 673-77.

Charney, E. (1972). Patient-doctor communication: Implications for the clinician. *Pediatric Clinics of North America*, 19, 263-79.

Cline, R. (1983). Interpersonal communication skills for enhancing physician-patient relationships. *Maryland State Medical Journal*, 32, 272-278.

Cline, R. & Cardosi, J. (1983). Interpersonal communication skills for physicians: A rationale for training. *Journal of Communication Therapy*, 2, 137-56.

Cody, M. (1982). A typology of disengagement strategies and an examination of the role intimacy, reaction to inequity, and relational problems play in strategy selection. *Communication Monographs*, 49, 148-70.

Courtwright, J., Millar, F., & Rogers-Millar, L. E. (1979). Domineeringness and dominance: Replication and expansion. *Communication Monographs*, 46, 179-92.

Cupach, W. & Spitzberg, B. (1981, February). *Relational competence: Measurement and validation*. Paper presented at the Western Speech Communication Association convention, Anaheim, CA.

Daly, M. & Hulka, B. (1975). Talking with the doctor 2. *Journal of Communication*, 25, 148-52.

Dickson-Markman, F. & Shern, D. (1984, May). *Social support and health: Is quantity as good as quality?* Paper presented at the International Communication Association convention, San Francisco.

DiMatteo, M. (1979). A social-psychological analysis of physician-patient rapport: Toward a science of the art of medicine. *Journal of Social Issues*, 35, 12-33.

Dindia, K. & Baxter, L. (1987). Strategies for maintaining and repairing marital relationships. *Journal of Social and Personal Relationships*, 4, 143-58.

Droge, D., Arntson, P. & Norton, R. (1981, May). *The social support function in epilepsy self help groups*. Paper presented at the International Communication Association convention, Minneapolis.

Duck, S. (1982). A typology of relationship disengagement and dissolution. In S. Duck (ed.), *Personal relationships 4: Dissolving personal relationships* (pp. 1-30). New York: Academic Press.

Duck, S. (1976). Interpersonal communication in developing acquaintance. In G. R. Miller (ed.), *Explorations in interpersonal communication* (pp. 127-47). Beverly Hills: Sage.

Fine, V., & Therrien, M. (1977). Empathy in doctor-patient relationship: Skill training for medical studies. *Journal of Medical Education, 52,* 752.

Fisher, B. A. & Drecksel, G. (1983). A cyclical model of developing relationships: A study of relational control interaction. *Communication Monographs, 50,* 67-78.

Fitzpatrick, M. & Best, P. (1979). Dyadic adjustment in traditional, independent, and separate relationships: A validation study. *Communication Monographs, 46,* 167-78.

Foley, R. & Sharf, B. (1981). The five interviewing techniques most frequently overlooked by primary care physicians. *Behavioral Medicine, 11,* 26-31.

Folger, J. & Poole, M. S. (1982). Relational coding schemes: The question of validity. In M. Burgoon (ed.), *Communication yearbook 5* (pp. 235-47). New Brunswick, NJ: Transaction.

Frank, L. (1961). Interprofessional communication. *American Journal of Public Health, 51,* 1798-1804.

Friedson, E. (1970). *Professional dominance: The social structure of medical care.* Chicago: Aldine.

Fuller, D. & Quesada, G. (1973). Communication in medical therapeutics. *Journal of Communication, 23,* 361-70.

Gibb, J. (1961). Defensive communication. *Journal of Communication, 3,* 141-48.

Golden, J. & Johnson, G. (1970). Problems of distortion in doctor-patient communication. *Psychiatry in Medicine, 1,* 127-49.

Gottlieb, B. (ed.). (1981). *Social networks and social support.* Beverly Hills: Sage.

Greenfield, S., Kaplan, S. & Ware, J. (1985). Expanding patient involvement in care. *Annals of Internal Medicine, 102,* 520-28.

Hawes, L. (1972a). Development and application of an interview coding system. *Central States Speech Journal, 23,* 92-99.

Hawes, L. (1972b). The effects of interviewer style on patterns of dyadic communication. *Speech Monographs, 39,* 114-23.

Hawes, L. & Foley, J. (1973). A Markov analysis of interview communication. *Speech Monographs, 40,* 208-19.

Kane, R. & Deuschle, K. (1967). Problems in doctor-patient communication. *Medical Care, 5,* 260-71.

Korsch, B., Gozzi, E. & Francis, V. (1968). Gaps in doctor-patient communication 1: Doctor-patient interaction and patient satisfaction. *Pediatrics, 42,* 855-71.

Korsch, B. & Negrete, V. (1972). Doctor-patient communication. *Scientific American, 227,* 66-74.

Krayer, K. & O'Hair, D. (1987, February). *A conversational analysis of reconciliation strategies.* Paper presented at the Western Speech Communication Association convention, Salt Lake City.

Kreps, G. (1988). The pervasive role of information in health and health care: Implications for health communication policy. In J. Anderson (ed.), *Communication yearbook 11* (pp. 238-76), Beverly Hills: Sage.

Kreps, G. (1986). Health communication and the elderly. *World Communication, 15,* 55-70.

Kreps, G. & Query, J. (1986, November). *Assessment and testing in the health professions.* Paper presented at the Speech Communication Association convention, Chicago.

Kreps, G. & Thornton, B. (1984, reissued 1992). *Health communication: Theory and practice.* Prospect Heights, IL: Waveland Press, Inc.

Lane, S. (1983). Compliance, satisfaction, and physician-patient communication. In R. Bostrum (ed.), *Communication yearbook 7,* (pp. 772-99). Beverly Hills: Sage.

Lane, S. (1982). Communication and patient compliance. In L. Pettegrew (ed.), *Straight talk: Explorations in Provider-Patient Interaction,* (pp. 59-69). Louisville, KY: Humana.

Lane, S. (1981, November). *Interpersonal situation: Empathic communication between medical personnel and patients.* Paper presented at the Speech Communication Association convention, Anaheim, California.

Ley, P. (1972). Comprehension, memory, and the success of communications with the patient. *Journal for Institutional Health Education,* 1972, 10, 23-29.

Maibach, E. & Kreps, G. (1986, September). *Communicating with patients: Primary care physicians' perspectives on cancer prevention, screening, and education.* Paper presented at the International Conference on Doctor-Patient Communication, Centre for Studies in Family Medicine, University of Western Ontario, London, Ontario, Canada.

Mechanic, D. (1972). *Public expectations and health care: Essays on the changing organization of health services.* New York: Wiley, 1972.

Millar, F. & Rogers, L. E. (1976). A relational approach to interpersonal communication. In G. R. Miller (ed.), *Explorations in interpersonal communication* (pp. 87-103). Beverly Hills, Sage.

Morse, B. & Piland, R. (1981). An assessment of communication competencies needed by intermediate-level health care providers: A study of nurse-patient, nurse-doctor, and nurse-nurse communication relationships. *Journal of Applied Communication Research,* 9, 30-41.

Myerhoff, B. & Larson, W. (1965). The doctor as cultural hero: The routinization of charisma. *Human Organization,* 24, 188-91.

Northouse, P. (1977). Predictors of empathic ability in an organizational setting. *Human Communication Research,* 3, 176-78.

O'Hair, D. & Krayer, K. (1987, May). *Reconciliation strategies in interpersonal communication relationships: A discovery and link to disengagement strategies.* Paper presented at the International Communication Association convention, Montreal.

O'Hair, D., O'Hair, M. J. & Kontas, G. (1985, November). *An examination of relational communication during physician and patient interactions.* Paper presented at the Speech Communication Association convention, Denver, Colorado.

Pacanowsky, M. & O'Donnell-Trujillo, N. (1982). Communication and organizational cultures. *Western Journal of Speech Communication,* 46, 115-30.

Parks, M. (1977). Relational communication: Theory and research. *Human Communication Research,* 3, 372-81.

Parks, M. & Adelman, M. (1983). Communication networks and the development of romantic relationships: An expansion of uncertainty reduction theory. *Human Communication Research,* 10, 55-79.

Pegels, C. (1980). *Health care and the elderly.* Rockville, MD: Aspen.

Pettegrew, L. & Thomas, R. C. (1978). Communication style differences in formal vs. informal therapeutic relationships. In B. Ruben (ed.), *Communication yearbook 2*, (pp. 523-38). New Brunswick, NJ: Transaction.

Pettegrew, L. (1977). An investigation of therapeutic communicator style. In B. Ruben (ed.), *Communication yearbook 1*, (pp. 593-604). New Brunswick, NJ: Transaction.

Powers, W. & Lowry, D. (1984). Basic communication fidelity: A fundamental approach. In R. Bostrum (ed.), *Competence in communication*, (pp. 57-71). Beverly Hills, CA: Sage.

Query, J. (1987). *A field test of the relationship between interpersonal communication competence, number of social supports, and satisfaction with the social support received by an elderly support group.* Unpublished master's thesis, Ohio University, Athens, Ohio.

Rogers, C. (ed.). (1967). *The therapeutic relationship and its impact.* Madison, WI: University of Wisconsin Press.

Rogers, C. (1957). The necessary and sufficient conditions of therapeutic personality change. *Journal of Consulting Psychology,* 21, 95-103.

Rogers, C. (1951). *Client-centered therapy.* Boston: Houghton Mifflin.

Rogers, L. E. & Farace, R. (1975). Analysis of relational communication in dyads: New measurement procedures. *Human Communication Research,* 1, 222-39.

Rossiter, C. (1975). Defining therapeutic communication. *Journal of Communication,* 25, 127-30.

Ruben, B. D. (1976). Assessing communication competency for intercultural adaptation. *Group and Organization Studies,* 1, 334-54.

Ruben, B. & Bowman, J. (1986). Patient satisfaction (part 1): Critical issues in the theory and design of patient relations training. *Journal of Health Care Education and Training,* 1, 1-5.

Ruben, B. & Kealey, D. (1979). Behavioral assessment of communication competency and the prediction of cross-cultural adaption. *International Journal of Intercultural Relations,* 3, 15-47.

Ruesch, J. (1963). The role of communication in therapeutic transactions. *Journal of Communication,* 13, 132-39.

Ruesch, J. (1961). *Therapeutic communication.* New York: Norton.

Ruesch, J. (1957). *Disturbed communication.* New York: Norton.

Ruesch, J. & Bateson, G. (1951). *The social matrix of psychiatry.* New York: Norton.

Salem, P. & Williams, M. L. (1984). Uncertainty and satisfaction: The importance of information in hospital communication. *Journal of Applied Communication Research,* 12, 75-89.

Spitzberg, B. (1984, May). *Relational competence: An empirical test of a conceptual model.* Paper presented at the International Communication Association convention, Boston.

Spitzberg, B. & Cupach, W. (1984). *Interpersonal communication competence.* Beverly Hills, CA: Sage.

Spitzberg, B. & Hecht, M. (1984). A component model of relational competence. *Human Communication Research,* 10, 575-600.

Stone, G. (1979). Patient compliance and the role of the expert. *Journal of Social Issues,* 35, 34-59.

Street, R. & Wiemann, J. (1987). Patients' satisfaction with physicians' interpersonal involvement, expressiveness, and dominance. In M. McLaughlin (ed.), *Communication yearbook* 10, (pp. 591-612). Newbury Park, CA: Sage.

Thompson, T. (1984). The invisible helping hand: The role of communication in the health and social service professions. *Communication Quarterly*, 32, 148-63.

Waitzkin, H. (1984). Doctor-patient communication: Clinical implications of social scientific research. *Journal of the American Medical Association*, 252, 17, 2441-46.

Waitzkin, H. & Stoekle, J. (1972). The communication of information about illness. *Advances in Psychosomatic Medicine, 8,* 180-215.

Waitzkin, H. & Stoekle, J. (1976). Information control and the micropolitics of health care: Summary of an ongoing research project. *Social Science and Medicine, 10,* 263-76.

Walker, H. (1973). Communication and the American health care problem. *Journal of Communication,* 23, 349-60.

Weg, R. (1975). Changing physiology of aging: Normal and pathological. In D. Woodruff & J. Birren (eds.), *Aging: Scientific perspectives and social issues,* (pp. 236-48). New York, Van Nostrand.

Wheeless, L. (1977). A follow-up study of the relationships among trust, disclosure and interpersonal solidarity. *Human Communication Research.* 4, 143-57.

Wheeless, L. (1976). Self disclosure and interpersonal solidarity: Measurement, validation, and relationships. *Human Communication Research,* 3, 47-61.

Wheeless, L. & Gratz, J. (1976). Conceptualization and measurement of reported self disclosure. *Human Communication Research,* 2, 338-46.

Wiemann, J. (1977). Evaluation and test of communication competence. *Human Communication Research,* 3, 195-213.

Worobey, J. L. & Cummings, H. W. (1984). Communication effectiveness of nurses in four relational settings. *Journal of Applied Communication Research,* 12, 128-41.

7

Health Care Providers and Consumers
Making Decisions Together
By Deborah Ballard-Reisch

Competent communication between health care practitioners and providers is the cornerstone of effective health care delivery (Kreps & Query, 1989; Roter, 1983). It affects patient satisfaction and compliance with treatment, and enhances patient recuperative abilities (Bertakis, 1977; Kreps & Query, 1989; Ley, 1983; Street & Wiemann, 1987). The characteristics of communication in the health provider-health consumer relationship are changing as a result of a growing trend in health care away from the traditional paternalistic model in which the physician prescribed and the patient complied (Ballard-Reisch, 1990) and toward a process of participative decision making in which the patient takes an active role in making health care decisions (see Ballard-Reisch, 1990; Katz, 1984; McNeil, Pauker, Sox, & Tversky, 1982). This paradigmatic shift away from the paternal and toward the participative necessitates a change in the modes of interaction in health contexts.

This article will 1) examine the nature of communication competence and therapeutic communication within the health care context, 2) explore the participative approach to health care decision making, 3) assess the roles and responsibilities of both health care consumers and providers within this framework and offer concrete steps that health care providers and consumers can take to communicate more effectively with one another.

Communication Competence and Therapeutic Communication

Competent communication within the health care context is "the ability to utilize interpersonal relations skills to elicit cooperation from, gather information from, and share health information with relevant individuals within the health

This article was written especially for this collection. The author is a faculty member of the Speech Communication Department at the University of Nevada, Reno.

care system" (Kreps & Query, 1989, p. 294). Therapeutic outcomes are enhanced by competent communication.

Duran (1983) and Spitzberg and Hecht (1984) identified communication competence as a gauge of effective communication. As a relational construct, the assessment of communication competence takes into account both the goals of the individuals and the relational demands of the situation. Duran and Zakahi (1983) view competence as the ability to perceive the needs of interpersonal relationships and to adapt one's interaction goals to meet these needs. The requirements of a dyadic approach to communication competence are (1) the requirements of both cognitive (ability to perceive) and behavioral (ability to adapt) skills; (2) adaptation of communication behaviors and goals; (3) the ability to perceive and adapt to the requirements of the situation; and (4) the assumption that perceptions of competence reside in the dyad (Duran, 1983).

It is the perspective of this author that within the health care context, competent communication is defined in terms of effective interaction geared toward therapeutic outcomes, what Fuller and Quesada (1973) refer to as satisfying relationships and positive health management. Therapeutic communication advances the successful management of illness or disease. As a result, it can occur between and among health care providers and consumers, members of a patient's support network and health care providers, patients and members of their support network, members of illness support groups and either patients or members of their support network. Communication among all these groups could be considered therapeutic if it leads to quality health management which enhances the goals of patient and provider in the health care context (Vaux, 1988). Kreps and Query (1989) refer to this social support as a form of "nonclinical therapeutic communication" (p. 297).

With an understanding of the goals of competent communication within the health care setting, it is appropriate to examine a model of participative decision making designed for the health care context which offers patients and practitioners a framework within which competent, therapeutic communication can occur.

Participative decision making in health care settings

The model of participative decision making developed by Ballard-Reisch (1990) proposes that decision making occurs in three phases within the health care process which is itself comprised of eight stages. This model is reproduced in Figure 1.

The three phases are the diagnostic phase; the exploration of treatment alternatives phase; and the treatment decision, implementation and evaluation phase.

1. *The Diagnostic Phase*

The diagnostic phase involves exploring the nature of the patient's condition and the characteristics and capabilities which affect the patient's ability

Figure 1 A Model of Participative Decision-Making in Physician-Patient Interaction

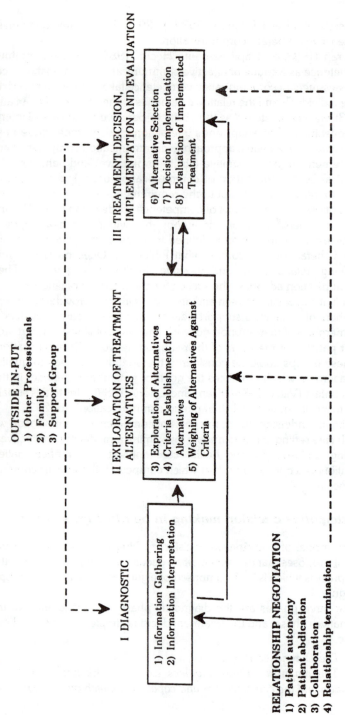

to deal with her/his condition. This process involves the collection of information by patient and practitioner so that both have a clear understanding of the nature of the patient's condition and its implications. Health care providers and patients will base initial perceptions on their prior beliefs, attitudes and values regarding illness and treatment (Weston & Brown, 1989). These perceptions and expectations will impact their initial interaction with one another and may ultimately affect the treatment selected as well as the patient's ability to deal with her/his condition.

It is also at this point that the relationship between the health care provider and patient is negotiated (Ballard-Reisch, 1990). *There are four relationship options which can be negotiated between practitioners and patients: patient autonomy, patient abdication, collaboration and relationship termination* (Ballard-Reisch, 1990).

Situation: Jennifer, age 6, was recently diagnosed as having leukemia. Her parents, Mr. and Mrs. Johnson are meeting with Dr. Carter, the physician in charge of the hospital's leukemia treatment program.

Dr. Carter's perspective: The hospital has one of the foremost leukemia treatment programs in the nation. They are currently in the middle of an extensive study of the effectiveness of four treatment protocols on recovery. Every new leukemic patient is randomly assigned to one of the four protocols. This is the most successful study in the history of leukemia research. Treatment decisions in this type of case must be made quickly for optimum outcomes. There is no time to waste. Dr. Carter will encourage Jennifer's parents to enroll her in the program immediately. Dr. Carter and the hospital are so sure of this program that they do not offer alternatives. There is not another leukemia treatment program in this region of the country.

Mr. Johnson's perspective: He is frightened. It is his desire to get Jennifer the best treatment available. He knows the hospital has a strong reputation. He has come to the meeting today intending to put his daughter's future in the doctor's hands.

Mrs. Johnson's perspective: She has taken a problem-solving approach to this situation. She wants to know all options available so that she can make the best decision for her daughter. She is surprised when Dr. Carter states that their only choice is to enter the pilot program. She inquires about other options and other programs as well as the success of the pilot program to date. She finds Dr. Carter nonresponsive as she continues to reinforce that the pilot program is the only option, that a decision must be made immediately, and that treatment alternatives are not available at this hospital.

Three of the provider/patient relationship alternatives occur on a continuum between patient control and practitioner control (see Figure 2).

At the practitioner control end of the continuum is patient abdication. Ballard-Reisch (1990) argues that this has been the most traditional model of physician-patient interaction in which the physician is ultimately responsible for decisions. Some of the reasons why patients choose to acquiesce in this kind of relationship are: the superior knowledge of the physician (or other health care provider), patient trust in the provider, a lack of willingness on the part of the patient to take responsibility for decision making, or the patient's feeling that s/he is not competent to make decisions. Mr. Johnson in the example above is operating out of this perspective. He feels that the physician has superior knowledge and abilities and that she is the best person to make decisions. Health care providers engage in this relationship alternative because it is the one with which they are most familiar, or because they feel that their superior knowledge and the lack of specialized knowledge on the part of the patient qualify them to make decisions. In the above example, Dr. Carter is operating from the superior knowledge perspective. She knows that the leukemia treatment program has been highly successful and that the decision to enroll in the program must be made immediately. There is no time to waste exploring options.

Some researchers (Caplan, 1988; Ingelfinger, 1980) contend that patient abdication is often an appropriate model as there are times when patients need someone else to make decisions for them, when time is short or when treatment alternatives do not exist. Communication patterns within this type of relationship involve the provider doing most of the talking, asking the majority of questions, choosing topics for discussion and interrupting the patient (Fisher, 1983; Frankel, 1984; West, 1984). The patient is often what Katz (1984) and Robinson and Whitfield (1985) refer to as passive and therefore, he/she is often reluctant to ask questions or express opinions.

Others advocate relationships somewhere between total patient dependence and total patient autonomy (see Caplan, 1988). This position represents the mid-point on the continuum; *collaboration.* In this type of relationship, *health*

Figure 2

Relational type continuum

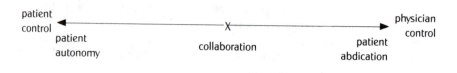

care provider and consumer both work actively, yet often unconsciously, through all three phases and eight stages of decision making, sharing information, negotiating perspectives and reaching a mutually satisfactory decision. A collaborative relationship has the most potential for effective communication and quality decision making. As Kreps and Query (1989) argue, competent communication between health care providers and consumers allows all parties to "gather and interpret pertinent information . . . encourages cooperation . . . and facilitates the sharing of relevant information necessary to accomplish health evaluation and maintenance" (p. 296). Patients interested in this type of relationship take responsibility for actively dealing with their health care problems by seeking information (Strickland, 1973). This is the perspective Mrs. Johnson is advancing in the above example. She wants to be effectively and actively involved in making quality decisions.

Health professionals who use the collaborative perspective view patients as having the right to participate actively in decisions which affect their health. This perspective is recommended by Babbie (1973); Ballard-Reisch (1990); Kreps (1988); and the President's Commission (1982) among others. In this relationship, communication behavior involves a more balanced approach to interaction, questioning, expressing opinions, and raising topics of concern. The process is marked by cooperation, negotiation and consensus. As noted in research on collaboration, this process is often time consuming (see Janis and Mann, 1977) and some medical decisions simply cannot wait.

The other end of the continuum is *patient autonomy.* This is the consumer model advocated by Slack (1977). In this relationship *the ultimate decision-making responsibility lies with the patient.* Patients operating in this framework are strongly oriented to their right to decide. They view themselves as purchasers of services and they will shop around until they receive a service with which they are satisfied. Providers who advocate this perspective believe in the rights of patients to self determination. This perspective is also advocated by Ley (1983) who argues that it eliminates many ethical concerns about compliance-induction attempts, particularly when: patients are presented with information about risks, and the effectiveness of various treatments; when they decide which, if any, treatment to try; when they have regular opportunities to withdraw from treatment. Slack (1977) also concludes that patients have the right to make informed medical decisions.

Communication in this type of relationship is the opposite of communication in the patient abdication model. Patients take an active role in health care discussions, asking questions, introducing topics of discussion, and expressing opinions. Provider communication varies according to her/his perspective on the situation. The provider may compete with the patient for dominance, displaying behavior consistent with the findings of Fisher (1983); Frankel (1984) and West (1984), or she/he may serve the function of an information giver, answering questions and giving advice.

The fourth relational option does not occur on the aforementioned continuum but is an alternative nonetheless. It is *relationship termination*. This relationship option can be an initial choice made during the diagnostic phase by the patient or practitioner if, for example, the practitioner is an inappropriate referral. In addition, it may arise out of dissatisfaction with the relationship type negotiated previously, or an inability on the part of the practitioner and patient to work together to the satisfaction of one or both parties.

Regardless of how active a role the patient desires to take in decision making, patient participation through open communication is fundamental to the effectiveness of the health care delivery process (Irwin, 1989). In addition, the negotiation of a relationship between patient and practitioner is not a static, one-time process. Although some patient-practitioner relationships are relatively stable across time, a relationship may vary along the continuum depending on the nature of the issues with which the provider and patient are faced at any given point in time.

Analysis: In the example provided at the beginning of this section, there is clearly a difference in the relational perspectives of Mrs. Johnson, Mr. Johnson and Dr. Carter. While Mr. Johnson and Dr. Carter are satisfied with a paternalistic relationship in which Dr. Carter is responsible for decisions and Mr. Johnson concurs, Mrs. Johnson is not comfortable with this arrangement and is likely to be frustrated and angry with Dr. Carter's seeming unwillingness to engage in a more collaborative relationship. Clearly, a relationship negotiation problem exists. How it is handled may well affect whether or not Jennifer's parents place her in the hospital's leukemia program as well as the success of Jennifer's treatment.

The diagnostic phase discussed in this section is, by far, the most time consuming, but the exploration of treatment alternatives phase and the treatment decision, implementation, and evaluation phase are of equal importance.

2. Exploration of Treatment Alternatives Phase

The exploration of treatment alternatives phase involves the generation of possible alternatives, the establishment of criteria for an effective decision and the process of weighing alternatives generated against criteria established. This phase is the most common place for the involvement of therapeutic and social support systems to begin, although they are important throughout the third phase as well. Patients should be encouraged to consult with other health care and auxiliary health care professionals as well as family, friends and clergy. Mobilizing a strong support system can have a significant impact on a patient's ability to cope with illness and disease (see Sullivan & Reardon, 1986).

The ability of health care practitioners (e.g. doctors, nurses) and auxiliary health care practitioners (e.g. social workers) to meet patient social support needs personally or to assist the patient's personal support network, including illness support groups, in meeting these needs can greatly assist the patient as she/he tries to cope with illness.

The exploration of alternatives involves the assessment of available treatment options and their costs and benefits. This involves reconciling the unique perspectives of the health care provider and the patient in the health care setting.

Situation: Dan is 61 years old. He suffers from rheumatoid arthritis, experiences a great deal of pain and has significant difficulty getting around on his own. His doctor strongly recommends a series of operations to replace Dan's hips and knees.

Physician's perspective: All conventional treatment regimens have been tried on Dan with little effect. Dan is currently undergoing drug therapy to control his pain. The longer Dan stays on drug therapy the less effective it becomes, the higher the doses he requests, the more serious the drug contraindications become. The only remaining alternative is surgery. Dan is in good health except for his arthritis. All signs indicate that he is an excellent candidate for surgery. The physician feels that the benefits of surgery, increased mobility and decreased pain, far outweigh the recuperative time Dan would require following surgery.

Patient's perspective: Dan is very independent. Although it is painful for him to get around, he is still mobile and self sufficient. He is terrified of surgery. He fears not only the procedure but the resultant convalescence as well. Giving up a year of his life to "feel better" does not seem a reasonable price to Dan. He feels an increase in the medication used to control his pain will meet his needs.

Clearly in the above example, the values and perspectives of the physician and patient are radically different. The physician's perspective, as is generally the case, is based upon the medical model which involves treating a condition; the patient's view is a highly personal approach to the health care situation in which quality of life issues are preeminent (Kassirer, 1983). The patient's personal view incorporates her/his beliefs, values and attitudes as well as the opinions of relevant individuals in her/his social support network (Albrecht & Adelman, 1987) which affect decisions about when to see a physician, feelings about treatment options and perceptions of illness in general (Weston & Brown, 1989).

Establishing a mutually agreed upon set of criteria for decision making involves the sharing of their beliefs, attitudes and values by both the health care practitioner and the patient and negotiating a perspective that is acceptable to all parties involved.

Analysis: Dan and his physician are operating out of very different perspectives. Their beliefs, attitudes and values concerning surgery and drug therapy are very different. The physician sees the likelihood of successfully managing a physical condition while Dan sees the potential for a costly convalescence and decreased quality of life for a year. Both must learn to see the other's perspective if they are to be able to arrive at a mutually satisfactory treatment option.

Once satisfactory negotiation has been completed, the weighing of alternatives against criteria will be principally an objective process of applying the criteria and, with appropriate modifications based upon negotiation, coming to a mutually satisfying treatment option.

3. *Treatment Decision, Implementation and Evaluation Phase*
The third phase is treatment decision, implementation and evaluation. This phase involves the selection of the treatment protocol, the implementation of the treatment regimen, and the evaluation of the effectiveness of treatment. This phase requires clear understanding and communication on the part of both patient and practitioner. The patient must be thoroughly prepared regarding the specifics of her/his treatment regimen, what to expect from treatment and what to do if and when unexpected outcomes occur. It is also necessary for the health care provider to understand the practicalities of how the treatment regimen will be integrated into the patient's life. Treatment cannot possibly be effective if it cannot be integrated with a minimum of discomfort.

Situation: Alan suffers from juvenile diabetes. His treatment protocol requires that he receive daily insulin shots. Alan has been on this program for 6 months. He finds the injections frightening and painful. He is only comfortable when his mother administers his shots. He becomes stressed and anxious and even hides or throws tantrums when anyone else attempts to give him insulin injections. He has broken syringes on three occasions when someone else has tried to give him shots. Recently, Mrs. Greene, Alan's mother, who is employed outside the home, has had her work schedule changed. She is now unavailable regularly when Alan's insulin injections need to be administered.

Nurse's perspective: Alan needs to have regular injections in order to control his diabetes. Something needs to be worked out to make this possible.

Alan's perspective: He is frightened. He doesn't know many of the doctors, nurses, and clinicians who have examined him, taken blood and given him shots in the past 6 months. He doesn't want strangers to hurt him anymore. Although the shots still hurt, Alan trusts his mother.

Mrs. Greene's perspective: Mrs. Greene must work in order to support her son. She had no choice regarding the schedule change and is feeling guilt and frustration over the situation. She is feeling guilt at not being able to be available to give Alan his shots as scheduled, and she is frustrated both with the seeming inflexibility of Alan's treatment schedule and Alan's inability to understand that others need to give him shots if she can't.

The health care provider needs to continually assess the patient's perceptions regarding treatment efficacy. Is the treatment working? What is the patient's perception of the treatment? Are there problems created by the regimen?

Analysis: The requirements of Alan's treatment regimen do not fit well into the realities of his life. His mother's work schedule and Alan's anxiety about receiving injections are having a detrimental effect on Alan's treatment regimen. Alternatives could center around assisting Alan in becoming comfortable with another care giver in the instances when his mother is unavailable to give his injections, changing Alan's eating schedule so that his mother can monitor his sugar level when she is home, or developing some mechanism (transportation to mother's office for example) to allow Alan and his mother to be together when injections need to be given.

The model of participative decision making advanced by Ballard-Reisch (1990) provides a framework within which health care providers and patients can work collaboratively to accomplish therapeutic outcomes (see Figure 1). The next section will outline the rights and responsibilities of both parties in concrete, communication-based terms in order to facilitate this process.

Provider and Patient Rights and Responsibilities

In the context of a collaborative approach to health care, the patient and the provider bear the responsibility for effective communication and quality decision making. As they are partners in the process of health management, both parties also possess certain rights and responsibilities. It is the perspective of this author that acknowledging the rights of the other and working to meet one's responsibilities with respect to personal needs, partner needs and the needs of the patient's social support network can lead to effective communication between patient and provider.

A number of writers, including Maurer (1986); Scully and Scully (1987), and the American Hospital Association (1972) have attempted to outline aspects of these rights and responsibilities. What follows in Figures 3 and 4 is a summary of some of their ideas on this topic.

Figure 3

Patient and health care provider rights

Patient rights:

Patients have the right to:
1. Participate in major decisions concerning their care.
2. Involve whomever they deem appropriate in the decision-making process.
3. Refuse treatment.
4. Receive as much information as they wish about their illness.
5. Receive adequate time with a health care provider to ask questions and express concerns about problems.
6. End their relationship with a health care provider.

Health Care Provider rights:

Health Care Providers have the right to:
1. Receive full patient disclosure of all pertinent information.
2. Take adequate time to gather and process the information necessary to effectively manage the patient's condition.
3. Receive prompt notification of worsening or change in symptoms, reactions to medications, or other health related concerns of their patients.
4. Be informed if their patients are or are not complying with treatment regimens.
5. Withdraw from the relationship with the patient as long as the professional assists the patient with a competent referral.

In short, patients have the right to be actively involved in the management of their health care from decision making regarding treatment acceptance or rejection to finding alternative health care providers if they so desire. Health care providers have the right to expect access to all pertinent information regarding a patient's condition, before, during, and after treatment.

Patients have a responsibility to engage in active information sharing with health care providers, to give all relevant information regarding treatment compliance and adverse effects of treatment regimens, and to ask questions when unclear about any facet of diagnosis or treatment. Health care providers have a responsibility to facilitate effective communication with patients, to involve them in discussion, and to allow adequate time for thorough information sharing.

Figure 4

Patient and health care provider responsibilities

Patient responsibilities:

Patients have the responsibility to:

1. Disclose all relevant information concerning their condition to the health care provider.
2. Prepare for consultations with health care providers.
3. Ask for clarification if information and explanations are unclear.
4. Ask questions.
5. Report all adverse affects of therapy, changes in condition or worsening symptoms.
6. Report any adverse affects of the patient's condition or therapy on patient's well-being or the patient's social support network.

Health care provider responsibilities:

Health Care Providers have a responsibility to:

1. Discuss thoroughly with the patient diagnosis, prognosis, testing and therapy.
2. Allow adequate time to listen to and understand the patient's perspective.
3. Present all generally accepted treatment alternatives, even if the provider does not recommend them.
4. Recommend to the patient the provider's perception of the best form of treatment and give justification.
5. Allow adequate time to answer patient questions and discuss patient concerns.
6. Provide adequate follow-up once treatment has been implemented.
7. Assist in obtaining relevant social services and rehabilitation services for the patient and her/his support network.

Summary and Conclusions

Competent therapeutic communication within the health care context is not a simple process. However, the movement toward participative decision making in health care offers the potential, as never before, for health care providers and consumers to interact effectively for health maintenance and management. The rights and responsibilities of health providers and consumers within this paradigm focus on the need for active participation and involvement in decision making. At best, this involves integrating the patient into decision making; at least, it involves the realization that the patient must take an active part in communication in order for both health care providers and consumers to work together toward therapeutic outcomes. How do health care providers and consumers begin?

With respect to consumers, a great deal of research has indicated that patients are uncomfortable or reluctant in asserting themselves in health care settings. A number of publications offer constructive suggestions for both increasing patient participation in health care decisions and dealing with some of the uncertainties and frustrations patients may face in this expanded role. This author's favorite is Thomas Scully, M.D. and Celia Scully's (1987) *Making medical decisions: How to make difficult medical and ethical choices for yourself and your family* published by Simon and Schuster. As Scully and Scully state, "the purpose of this book is to help you avoid intimidation and to enhance the dialogue which must take place if you are going to protect yourself and your loved ones, get the best medical treatment available, and become an equal partner in biomedical negotiations in which, traditionally, health care professionals have had the upper hand" (p. 33). Of particular interest is their list of "questions to ask for informed consent" on p. 70-71. They conclude that patients should read about their "condition, its diagnosis and treatment" (p. 71) and if they have doubts about their physicians' recommendations, patients should ask additional questions. If they are still not satisfied, they should obtain a second opinion. They suggest a patient should "become an informed consumer" (p. 71).

A second volume is Janet M. Maurer, M.D.'s (1986) *How to talk to your doctor* published by Simon and Schuster. Maurer states "this is a handbook for patients. It is designed to educate them about their medical problems. It is meant to foster a cooperative effort between patients and doctors, because it is the most positive approach and the most likely to improve health care" (p. 11).

With respect to health care providers, research has already indicated that communication techniques can be effectively used to facilitate communication with patients. Steps the physician can take to improve patient understanding and the likelihood of compliance with treatment decisions include previewing information to be given, dividing information into categories (Ley, 1979; Ley, Bradshaw, Eaves, & Walker, 1973), repeating information (Greenberg et al., 1984; Ley, 1979), and questioning the patient about instructions to assess understanding (Bertakis, 1977). In addition, the physician must keep in mind that s/he is not just dealing with an illness per se, s/he is dealing with a unique individual within whose life an illness has been made manifest. Therefore, listening to the patient's perspective and assisting with the integration of the illness and/or treatment into the patient's life can prove beneficial to the advancement of therapeutic outcomes.

Finally, research has found that the social support network of the patient can have a significant impact on patient coping and, ultimately, the success or failure of treatment. The support network needs further attention, both through inclusion in the decision-making process, where deemed appropriate by the patient, and integration into the health care network including access to counselors, therapists, and illness support groups.

The goal of health communication is therapeutic outcomes. The process of participative decision making offers a framework within which the dynamics of provider and consumer needs as well as the impact of the patient's social support network can be assessed so that competent communication and therapeutic outcomes can be achieved.

References

Albrecht. T. & Adelman, M. (1987). *Communicating social support.* Newbury Park, CA: Sage.

American Hospital Association. (1972). A patient's bill of rights. In Scully, T. and Scully, C. *Making medical decisions,* (pp. 342-44). New York: Simon & Schuster, Inc.

Babbie, S. (1973). *Medical communication requirements.* Springfield, VA: U. S. Pacific.

Ballard-Reisch, D. (1990). A model of participative decision making for physician-patient interaction. *Health Communication,* 2(2), 91-104.

Bertakis, K. (1977). The communication of information from physician to patient: A method for increasing patient retention and satisfaction. *Journal of Family Practice,* 5, 217-22.

Caplan, A. L. (1988). Informed consent and provider-patient relationships in rehabilitation medicine. *Archives of Physical Medicine and Rehabilitation,* 69, 312-17.

Duran, R. (1983). Communicative adaptability: A measure of social communicative competence. *Communication Quarterly,* 31, 320-26.

Duran, R. & Zakahi, W. (April, 1983). *Competence or style: What's in a name?* Paper presented at the annual Eastern Communication Association conference, Ocean City, MD.

Fisher, S. (1983). Doctor talk/patient talk: How treatment decisions are negotiated in doctor/patient communication. In S. Fisher & A. Todd (eds.), *The social organization of doctor-patient communication* (pp. 135-57). Washington, DC: Center for Applied Linguistics.

Frankel, R. M. (1984). From sentence to sequence: Understanding the medical encounter through microinteractional analysis. *Discourse Processes,* 7, 135-70.

Fuller, D. & Quesada, G. (1973). Communication in medical therapeutics. *Journal of Communication,* 23, 361-70.

Greenberg, L. W., Jewett, L. S., Glick, R. S., Champion, L. A., Leiken, S. L., Althiere, M. F., & Lipnick, R. N. (1984). Giving information for a life threatening diagnosis. *American Journal of Diseases of Children,* 138, 649-53.

Ingelfinger, F. J. (1980). Arrogance. *New England Journal of Medicine,* 303, 1507-11.

Irwin, H. (February, 1989). A competence model for interpersonal health communication. Paper presented at the International Health Communication Conference, Monterey, CA.

Janis, I. & Mann, L. (1977). *Decision making: A psychological analysis of conflict, choice, and commitment.* New York, NY: The Free Press.

Kassirer, J. P. (1983). Adding insult to injury: Usurping patient prerogatives. *New England Journal of Medicine,* 308, 898-901.

Katz, J. (1984). *The silent world of doctor and patient.* London: Free Press.

Kreps, G. L. (1988). The pervasive role of information in health and health care: Implications for health communication policy. In J. A. Anderson (ed.), *Communication yearbook* (Vol. 11, pp. 238-76) Beverly Hills: Sage.

Kreps, G. L. & Query, J. L. (1989). Health communication and interpersonal competence. In G. M. Phillips & J. T. Woods (eds.), *SCA 75th anniversary commemorative volume.* (pp. 293-323). Carbondale: Southern Illinois University Press.

Ley, P. (1983). Patient's understanding and recall in clinical communication failure. In D. Pendleton & J. Hasler (eds.), *Doctor patient communication* (pp. 89-107). New York: Academic.

Ley, P. (1979). The psychology of compliance. In D. Oborne, M. Gruneberg & R. Eiser (eds.), *Research in psychology and medicine* (Vol. 2, pp. 221-34). London: Academic.

Ley, P., Bradshaw, P. W., Eaves, D., & Walker, C. M. (1973). A method for increasing patient's recall of information presented by doctors. *Psychology of Medicine, 3,* 2217-30.

Maurer, J. M. (1986). *How to talk to your doctor: The questions to ask.* New York: Simon & Schuster, Inc.

McNeil, B., Pauker, S., Sox, H., & Tversky, A. (1982). On the elicitation of preferences for alternative therapies. *New England Journal of Medicine, 306,* 1259-62.

President's Commission for the Study of Ethical Problems in Medicine and Biomedical and Behavioral Research. (1982). *Making health care decisions* (Vol. 1). Washington DC: U. S. Government Printing Office. (NTIS No. PB83-236711)

Robinson, E. J. & Whitfield, M. J. (1985). Improving the efficiency of patients' comprehension monitoring: A way of increasing patients' participation in general practice consultations. *Social Science Medicine, 21,* 915-19.

Roter, D. L. (1983). Physician/patient communication: Transmission of information and patient effects. *Maryland State Medical Journal, 32,* 260-65.

Scully, T. and Scully, C. (1987). *Making medical decisions: How to make difficult medical and ethical choices for yourself and your family.* New York: Simon & Schuster, Inc.

Slack, W. V. (1977). The patient's right to decide. *The Lancet, 2,* 240.

Spitzberg, B. and Hecht, M. (1984). A component model of relational competence. *Human Communication, 10,* 575-99.

Street, R. L., Jr. & Wiemann, J. M. (1987). Patient satisfaction with physicians' interpersonal involvement, expressiveness, and dominance. In M. L. McLaughlin (ed.), *Communication yearbook* (Vol. 10, pp. 591-612). Newbury Park, CA: Sage.

Strickland, B. (September, 1973). *Locus of control: Where have we been and where are we going?* Paper presented at the American Psychological Association, Montreal, Canada.

Sullivan, C. F. & Reardon, K. K. (1986). Social support satisfaction and health locus of control: Discriminators of breast cancer patients' styles of coping. In M. L. McLaughlin (ed.), *Communication yearbook* (Vol. 9, pp. 707-22). Beverly Hills: Sage.

Vaux, A. (1988). *Social support.* New York: Praeger Publishers.

West, C. (1984). *Routine Complications.* Bloomington: Indiana University Press.

Weston, W. W. & Brown, J. B. (1989). The importance of patients' beliefs. In M. Stewart & D. Roter, (eds.), *Communicating with medical patients.* (pp. 77-85). Newbury Park: Sage Publications.

CHAPTER
4

Group Communication in Health Care

Groups are a critical operational level in the modern health care system, since specialized groups (such as health care teams, peer support groups, quality circles, ethics committees, and group medical practices) are used in modern health care to gather, process, and disseminate relevant health information, as well as to perform many complex health care goals through the coordinated efforts of group members (Kreps, 1988; Thornton, 1978). Group communication is the primary means by which group member coordination and goal attainment is accomplished. For example, communication enables individual group members to establish and maintain important group roles (such as leadership); communication is used to manage group conflicts; communication is the means by which social support is provided among group members; and communication is the primary mechanism for facilitating effective group decision making.

81

Groups depend on the development of networks of interpersonal relationships between members to elicit cooperation and coordination within the group. Group members learn to perform both task and maintenance (socioemotional) roles to facilitate the accomplishment of formal group goals and the preservation of effective working relationships within the group. For example, the emergence and expression of the leadership role is a critical factor in group performance, accomplished through the use of persuasive communication by influential group members. Communication is the means by which leadership is expressed. Effective leaders use communication to provide group members with both rationale and direction for accomplishing group goals. The most effective leaders provide their followers with attractive and motivating visions that describe group goals and values and explain the need for accomplishing group tasks. Charismatic leaders provide members with symbolic visions that encourage personal identification with the group and its mission, motivating high performance, cooperation, and teamwork among group members.

Conflict is an inevitable part of group interaction. Since all individuals perceive reality idiosyncratically, group members are likely to disagree about and struggle over the efficacy of different group activities and goals. Such conflict is potentially productive to group performance when it focuses on substantive issues and enables group members to examine alternatives before making important decisions. Substantive conflict reduces the threat of groupthink, where groups make risky decisions without carefully examining alternatives. Conflict can be destructive when it emphasizes affective (personal attributes of members) issues, alienating members from one another and complicating group decision making. Since conflict is expressed through group member communication, strategic communication can be used to contain and direct conflict. Kreps and Thornton (1992), for example, suggest the development of ethical conflict strategies to effectively manage group conflict to maximize the productive aspects and minimize the destructive aspects of conflict.

This section of the book examines several of the important roles performed by groups in modern health care and illustrates the powerful influences of communication on group performance. The first reading was originally published in the *Medical Laboratory Observer*. The author, Ed Roseman, explains the importance of cooperation between different groups of professionals within health care organizations. In highly stressful health care settings, bad experiences, value differences, status inequalities, competition and misunderstandings can cause clashes between different groups. Roseman describes step-by-step procedures for facilitating intergroup cooperation in health care.

The second reading, by Edward Madara, is an article concerning the development of self-help groups that was originally published in the journal *Social Policy*. Edward Madara is director of the New Jersey and the American Self-Help Clearinghouses at St. Clares-Riverside Medical Center, Denville, New Jersey 07834. The American Clearinghouse provides contacts for national and model self-help groups through its information line (201) 625-7101 and its *Self-Help Sourcebook* directory printed biennially. He describes how clearinghouses work to increase the use and development of relevant self-help groups. These clearinghouses provide consumers with information about local self-help groups and help people who need support and information concerning health issues not served by existing local groups establish their own groups. Have you ever participated in a self-help group? Can you identify any local self-help groups that serve the city where you live?

The final reading in this chapter, written specifically for this book by Barbara Thornton, describes the roles and functions of ethics committees in modern health care organizations. This reading examines this new small group phenomenon in health care and its relationship to health communication. As you read, try to identify the similarities and differences between group communication in ethics groups and the communication in traditional health care teams such as emergency room (E.R.) or operating room (O.R.) teams. What do ethics committees do that these other teams rarely take the time to do? In Chapter 8, we will examine the importance of communicating about ethical issues as a further attempt to tie together the important issues of health communication and ethics.

Kreps, G. L. (1988). The pervasive role of information in health and health care: Implications for health communication policy. In J. Anderson (ed.), *Communication Yearbook 11* (pp. 238-76). Newbury Park, CA: Sage.

Kreps, G. L. & Thornton, B. C. (1992). *Health Communication: Theory and Practice* 2nd edition. Prospect Heights, IL: Waveland Press.

Thornton, B. C. (1978). Health care teams and multimethodological research. In B. Ruben (ed.), *Communication Yearbook 2* (pp. 538-53). New Brunswick, NJ: Transaction Press.

8

How to Overcome Intergroup Conflict

By *Ed Roseman*

"You can't trust them. They're the enemy."

Ever hear that comment? Unfortunately, such negative stereotypes are common at hospitals. Physicians think nurses are inferior, nurses say technologists are rude, and technologists think that physicians are inconsiderate. Even within the laboratory itself preconceived notions exist: Other techs may look down on, say, phlebotomists. And so it goes, a series of sweeping bad raps.

Negative feelings held by one group toward another limit interaction and communication. This information gap may spawn job errors.

Even when the groups interact, they read between the lines and listen selectively. Distortion and inaccuracies occur. Unfortunately, once this kind of adversary relationship develops, it tends to persist and worsen over time. Newcomers get the word on how to deal with "those people." Every incident is magnified:

"Internal medicine complained again that Stat reports take too long. We'll never be able to satisfy them. I don't know what they want from us."

We all experience natural confrontations that can lead to adversarial relationships. These confrontations fall into five general categories. Let's take a look at them:

- **Bad experiences**. Perhaps your group made an error or was legitimately late with a Stat order because of conflicting demands. For real or imagined reasons, your group appeared to be uncooperative. The incident is blown out of proportion. Each side believes it can do no wrong and the other can do no right.

- **Value differences**. Various groups often use the same "facts" differently. For example, a physician requests a Stat test; his patient's symptoms are

Reprinted by permission of the Medical Economics Company, Inc. from the *Medical Laboratory Observer* 12 (June 1980): 41-44. Dr. Roseman, at the time of this writing, was a member of the Medical Laboratory Observer Editorial Advisory Board and president of Answers & Insights, a management consulting firm in East Brunswick, NJ.

severe, and the diagnosis is unclear. He transmits his sense of urgency to the nursing staff when he asks for the results as soon as possible. The nursing staff wants to comply with the physician's request and worries about the consequences of any delay.

Your group in the laboratory must manage a total workload, including special requests. Heavy demands bear in from all sides. You try to balance the work orders. When you can't satisfy the nurse's rush request, and she in turn must face an angry physician, it's not surprising that friction results.

- **Status inequalities**. In a professional environment, where position derives from educational background, high-status employees often throw their weight around. For example, physicians may pull rank to get special treatment. This causes resentment among lower-status groups.

- **Competition**. Groups compete for money, attention, or occasionally just for the sake of competing. Whatever the issues, small or large, one group aims to gain an advantage over another.

In a laboratory planning to expand its crowded quarters, for example, the lab manager asked each department head to submit a request for needed additional space. The resultant jockeying for space completely disrupted work and alienated departments that had formerly worked well together.

- **Misunderstandings**. Adversaries keep their distance, communicate minimally, and avoid discussing grievances. Minor irritations accumulate under these circumstances. Then they escalate into more serious problems.

When distance grows between coworkers, so do misunderstandings. When the other group does something you don't like you assume they're deliberately provoking you.

For example, the day staff in a laboratory resented the mess and the leftover work it constantly inherited from the night crew. As a result, the two groups feuded continually. Yet the real problem was understaffing of the night crew. They didn't have time to clean up properly or complete their workload.

Even when groups recognize that natural confrontations exist and can bring on adversarial dealings, they rarely do anything to strengthen the relationship. They don't get to know each other better or work toward mutual understanding. They seldom respond to the other party's needs and generally tend to deal with each other destructively rather than constructively.

Intergroup conflict is not inevitable. The five-step program outlined as follows can help your group improve its relationships with others:

- **Foster personal understanding**. Schedule a meeting between the two groups in conflict. Once they have assembled, tell them that you want to improve overall effectiveness. Instruct each group to go into a separate workroom and answer these questions:

How do we view the other group?

How do we think they see us?

How do we see ourselves?

What would we like them to do more of, less of, the same?

Answers should be candid and present both the consensus and range of opinion. Some group members may have strong feelings, for example, while others may not really care. Group members should also explain the origin of their feelings and indicate how long they have held them.

When they're ready, reassemble both groups. Then have representatives deliver each side's detailed answers.

These reports form the basis for a constructive discussion, focusing on what the groups can do together to improve joint effectiveness. Be sure to keep the emphasis on the current situation instead of trying to justify or defend past actions.

This meeting, called an "organizational mirror," is the first step in combating the negative stereotypes each group has of the other. Members of one group know exactly how those in the other see them, and they can now work together to strengthen their relationships.

- **Plan for more and better communication**. This guarantees that members of different groups get to know each other and appreciate each other's problems. Here are some ideas you might consider:

1) Exchange reports covering department news, current workload, special difficulties, and anything else that might help others understand your group's unique working environment.

2) Distribute regular feedback reports that describe what you'd like the other group to do more of, less of, and the same.

3) Organize methods-improvement or work-simplification teams, allowing members of different groups to work together on planning and problem solving.

- **Manage boundaries**. Certain members of a work group have more opportunity to interact with other groups. As a result, they become the group in the eyes of outsiders, and bear a certain responsibility. If they do something positive, it reflects well on their whole group; if they do something negative, it reflects badly on their group.

These special group members can advise their colleagues on ways to achieve intergroup cooperation.

- **Build trust**. Always make sure your group's intentions are known. This way, you avoid experiencing the unpleasant and common confrontation, "Why didn't you tell me you were going to do that?"

A group wins trust when its members take care not to harm another group through personal attacks, embarrassing actions or threats. This trust develops when you consistently demonstrate cooperation and support.

- **Create goodwill.** When you work on behalf of another group without any expectation of immediate return, you build goodwill.

Instead of waiting to be asked for example, volunteer assistance. If another group has problems, show genuine concern about the group members and the difficulties they are experiencing. In whatever concessions your group can make, be reasonable and flexible.

Most important, whenever your plans affect another group consider the consequences. Ask yourself, "Will I hurt them?" "Would alternative steps cause less harm without compromising my objectives?"

Your goodwill to other groups will pay off in the end. A common theme underlying the entire five-step process is: Act constructively with others, trying to satisfy their needs, and they will follow your example.

No group can afford to alienate itself from other groups. We function in an interdependent environment: We need them, and they need us. By actively cooperating with others, we can improve intergroup relationships and strengthen effectiveness.

9

Supporting Self-Help
A Clearinghouse Perspective

By *Edward J. Madara*

Self-help clearinghouses represent one of the most exciting and innovative forms of human services today. Over 40 self-help centers have been created across the country over the last decade, each of which has been finding new and different ways to increase the awareness, use, and development of self-help groups in their communities. These clearinghouses also serve as bridges for increasing communication and collaboration between the self-help and professional communities. Clearinghouses demonstrate, through their work, some of the possibilities that exist for any organization to promote and collaborate with self-help groups in better meeting people's health and human needs. Our experience in New Jersey is one example.

At our Medical Center, it all began with just a one-page list that included contacts for some two dozen local self-help groups. We had compiled it because several hospital staff often asked for such "hard-to-find" community resources and reported how patients were so very grateful to learn of them; groups were meeting many emotional and practical needs that professionals could not address. As the list was circulated, it grew to nearly 70 groups.

The listing was published as the first such directory in the state, under a grant from Hoffman LaRoche, Inc. It included national groups that had no local chapters, so people could see what new groups might be started. We had observed a powerful "demonstrational effect;" lay persons were much more likely to start a new self-help group in their community if they could be encouraged with evidence that others had started a similar group elsewhere. We linked people with all the related national or model groups that we could identify, so they wouldn't have to "reinvent the wheel." As an example, we had numerous callers requesting information on groups for survivors of suicide,

Reprinted with permission from *Social Policy* 16 (1987): 28-29. The author, at the time of this writing, was director of the New Jersey Self-Help Clearinghouse and the American Self-Help Clearinghouse.

but none existed in the state. Finally, we sent callers material from a model group in the Midwest. One woman called back in tears, explaining that the material had shown her how starting such a group could "provide meaning to a meaningless act."

As more lay people called seeking a group, if there was no local group to refer them to, we began to ask, "Would you be interested in joining with others to form a group?" For those who said "yes," we recorded their names so we could link them with the next caller who might be similarly interested in developing that type of group. Like rubbing two sticks of wood together to start a fire, such linkages often resulted in new groups. We began to realize that, with a little encouragement and support, some of these "help seekers" could be readily transformed into "resource developers" who started new groups.

We have found that one of the most appropriate roles that any professional can take in helping a group is that of a consultant — one who offers advice and counsel, but does not assume responsibility for actual decision making or leadership. The professional remains, as Dr. Leonard Borman once said, "on tap, not on top."

In 1980, funding was provided by the State Division of Mental Health and Hospitals to extend our services to the entire state using toll-free phone lines and developing a computer system that would include local, state, and national databases. We anticipated that toll-free telephone consultation would not only be cost-effective, but would decrease the risk of the consultee becoming too dependent upon the professional consultant. Since that time, we have assisted in the development of over 420 new groups.

Clearinghouses have helped to start groups that have developed into state or national foundations. We should recognize that the seeds for the development of many long-standing health foundations, societies, and agencies dealing with specific illnesses historically have first taken the form of self-help groups. The cycle continues today as improved medical technology and research increases the survival for previously life-threatening disorders, while also continuing to identify new specialty disorders.

In 1984, one caller who was blind educated us to the need for the development of special self-help groups for persons who were losing their sight. Working with him, we wrote a proposal that provided him with a driver, staff, and a position at the clearinghouse. John Dehmer and his staff have thus far started over 30 self-help groups across the state for persons who are visually impaired or adjusting to blindness. A similar clearinghouse program developed groups for former mental patients and for families of the mentally ill. Coalitions of both groups now receive their own state funding for their respective statewide operations. In current development work, the clearinghouse continues to use self-help group representatives as paid part-time advisors for consultation and training.

The clearinghouse currently helps over 10,000 callers a year with referrals, over a third of whom are professionals. A state directory is published each year, along with newsletters and various how-to materials. Conferences, and workshops are held throughout the year, where professionals and self-help leaders learn from one another. Foundation-funded grants have included the creation and distribution of Tel-Med tapes on self-help to every hospital in New Jersey, and the publication of a national directory of groups.

There is a Great Need for Learning

It was Marie Killilea, speaking at one of our New Jersey conferences, who wisely counselled us that "the first thing that professionals have to learn about self-help groups is that there is something to learn." While professionals have become more aware of the value of self-help groups, few understand the underlying principles of self-determination and empowerment that contribute to the very life and success of these groups. By understanding these principles, we can have a better appreciation for how to form partnerships without compromising the essential nature of self-help.

I believe the most important principle to respect is that of self-determination. Several years ago I asked Dr. Agnes Hatfield, a researcher who is one of the founders of the National Alliance for the Mentally Ill, what she felt was the most important factor that contributed to the vitality of a successful self-help group. Her reply was in one word, ownership, a sense of ownership on the part of the members. To the extent that members recognize the group as "theirs," they will invest time and effort in making the group work and keeping it focused on their needs. But to the extent that they perceive the group to be owned by someone else — either a professional, a dominating leader, or an agency — they will tend to step back and let those responsible for it do the work. In negotiating any partnership, a true sense of equality and mutual respect for each others' values and knowledge is needed, whether it be experiential or professional knowledge.

Some groups are advocacy oriented, reflecting a healthy skepticism of our health care delivery system and helping to make health care more responsive to consumer needs. Other self-help groups work in prevention by reducing stress in general, as well as through educational programs. Other groups supplement and "humanize" treatment services by serving as an adjunct to treatment or providing support and help not available within the professional milieu. Finally, groups provide after-care services that would reduce recidivism, institutionalization, and readmissions to the health care system.

Hopeful Areas for the Future

The media provides our clearinghouse with the most referrals. For example, one call came from a woman who had been sexually abused by her father 40 years earlier but had never had the courage to discuss it with anyone, neither

her husband nor her counselors, until she saw a television program depicting an incest survivor's self-help group, and she realized for the first time that she wasn't alone. Clearly the media have a tremendous power to inform people about self-help. From promoting weekly newspaper listings of groups, to developing public service announcements, we can do much to maximize these media resources.

High-tech telephone and home computer conferencing systems have permitted an increasing number of self-help groups to "meet" over great distances via new telecommunication systems. Health care and other agencies can play a role in making this technology more available to self-help groups for outreach to rural areas, and for the participation of persons who are unable to leave their homes or hospital beds. Our clearinghouse has hosted several national self-help meetings of persons with disabilities and rare illnesses who participated from their homes, some of whom went on to form a national foundation for Ehlers Danlos Syndrome. Electronic communication will increase the linkage of people, ideas, and concerns, while providing many innovative ways for people to find and develop the mutual aid and support they need.

Local self-help clearinghouses and resource centers, which serve almost half the country, have their own stories to tell about partnerships that they helped create. The International Network for Mutual Help Centers, an association of self-help resource centers that was formed in 1985, serves as a forum for the development and exchange of these and other ideas that support the philosophy and practice of self-help mutual aid. Through the work of its four representatives, it was honored to have cooperated in planning this workshop and hopes its members may be of service in making the workshop recommendations a reality.

We all have a profound realization of the incredible potential of self-help groups. We recognize that, at the very least, more must be done to make professionals aware of these resources so that more people find the support and help they need. Just as it would be unethical for a physician to withhold medication that he or she knew would help a patient, with the increasing amount of research that indicates the value of social support, we now must ask ourselves if there isn't a similar obligation to provide a patient with a referral to a self-help group, knowing that it can both reduce suffering and promote recovery or rehabilitation.

10

The Ethics Committee As a Small Group

By Barbara C. Thornton

Ethics committees are interdisciplinary small groups, usually in hospital or institutional settings that assist individuals or institutions in addressing the ethical dilemmas of health care. While it is sometimes difficult to determine what is or is not an ethical problem, issues of what one ought or ought not to do or what is good or bad for the patients are generally accepted as matters of ethical concern. For example, whether to administer one of two equally effective and cost-equivalent medications is not an ethics question. Whether to violate the confidentiality of a patient is, however, clearly a moral issue.

Ethical decisions were traditionally made until the 1950s by the physician for the patient because almost all of these decisions were seen as primarily medical. After the 1950s when the doctrine of informed consent became legal and morally advisable, some physicians began to include patients in the decision making. By the 1980s, with the widespread acceptance of technological solutions to medical dilemmas, patients and physicians were often found to disagree about moral answers to medical questions and the ethics committee was developed in part to assist in advising health care providers and institutions about these difficult issues.

Advocates of ethics committees stress the importance of interdisciplinary opinions regarding moral dilemmas as well as the reasoned reflection that diverse members can provide. Committees can be particularly helpful in certain complicated cases. If the alternatives are controversial, an advisory opinion by a group can be helpful to the physician, the patient and/or the family. Additionally, a group of people focusing specifically on moral issues in health care institutions raises the consciousness of the staff and the community.

Ethics committees are rooted in several major historical developments. In Seattle, Washington, treatment committees were established in the 1960s to

This article was written especially for this collection. Dr. Thornton is a faculty member at the University of Nevada-Reno in the Department of Community Health Sciences, and is an active participant in the field of bioethics as well as health communication.

review the cases of patients who were medically qualified for dialysis. Decisions needed to be made because there were not enough dialysis machines. These committees were disbanded when the government provided the funds to treat more patients. The committees had been criticized for using social worth rather than ethically based criteria for making their decisions (Ross, 1986).

In 1972 a judicial opinion in the Karen Quinlan case by the New Jersey Supreme Court recommended that a committee be consulted together with physicians to determine if Quinlan (23 years old and in a persistent vegetative state) should be kept on a respirator as her physician recommended or whether the respirator should be turned off as her parents wished (Ross, 1986). The push toward committees was furthered by the Baby Doe cases and the government's response (Cranford and Doudera, 1984).

Although an ethics committee did not ultimately make the decision in the Quinlan case, it was the discussion surrounding this case that encouraged the formation of such committees. The idea of the ethics committee is certainly a part of current health care. In 1982, a survey of ethics committees indicated that approximately 10% of hospitals had such committees. By 1988 it was estimated that 60% of hospitals with over 200 beds had them and nursing homes, dialysis centers and home health care services were beginning to form them (Cohen, 1988).

Committees generally range in size from five to forty, thus fitting the communication criteria of a small group. Estimates indicate that a third or more of the members of a committee will generally be specialists in areas where problems occur, a third will be nurses who are often administrators and the other third will include social workers, chaplains, patient representatives and lawyers. Often hospital administrators or their staff will serve in an ex-official capacity. (Bosford, 1986). Whether patients, families or other laypersons without special expertise should serve on committees is still a matter of debate (Rues and Weaver, 1989).

Maryland, the first state to enact legislation requiring all hospitals in its jurisdiction to have committees called Patient Care Advisory Committees, requires that a physician, a nurse not involved in the care of the patient in question, a social worker and a chief executive officer of the hospital be included (Hollinger, 1989).

Institutional ethics committees sometimes serve as committees for the institution as a whole and undertake to discuss and consult regarding infant care cases, while other organizations have separate infant bioethics committees. Both kinds of committees were recommended where appropriate by the President's Commission on Medical Ethics, particularly in the volume which addressed deciding whether to waive treatment (President's Commission, 1983). The infant review committees have also been supported and encouraged by federal child abuse regulations.

Ethics committees have three generally recognized functions: to educate, to assist in the formulation of policy and to advise on cases when asked to do so. Ideas for education, policy issues and cases are brought to the committee from many sources. Administrators usually ask for the policy formulation and sometimes the educational assistance. Cases are generally suggested by physicians although nurses are increasingly using the ethics committees when they are concerned about patient treatment. Some committees advertise their services to patients and their families, others do not (Bosford, 1986; Cranford & Doudera, 1984; and Ross, 1986).

The first and most utilized function of the committees is that of education. Most committees seek to educate themselves regarding ethical issues and to seek some understanding of how philosophy and other disciplines have impacted medical ethics. Some committees have libraries and share readings; others frequently call on consultants from disciplines such as philosophy to assist in their education about ethical concerns.

The second function of committees is policy making. The recent focus within the United States on termination of treatment and death and dying issues has forced institutions to begin to develop policies on resuscitation, hydration and nutrition, and other critical areas. The ethics committee is increasingly given the responsibility of developing such policies in the belief that their interdisciplinary composition can adjudicate the many views regarding such issues. This is not always an easy task. Ruth Macklin discusses the difficulty her institution had in developing a policy regarding pregnant Jehovah Witness patients and blood transfusions (Macklin, 1987). Most recently, there has been some heated discussion as to whether ethics committees should be called upon to assist in making policy on cost containment issues, since cost containment clearly has a moral dimension when policy makers decide who should or should not be treated (Brock, 1990).

The third and most controversial task of the committees is that of case review, both proactive and retroactive. Few committees, if any, are given the authority to decide an ethical matter, but they are often called upon to discuss cases and assist the physician and sometimes the patient and family in making an ethical decision. Committees become particularly important when the physician and the family disagree about treatment (Smith, 1989). Some committees also set aside time to discuss past cases in order to standardize procedures for the future. Many physicians and commentators on ethics committees still see decision-making as belonging primarily, if not exclusively, to the physician and the patient. While they will accept the education and policy functions of committees, they draw the line at case review (Siegler, 1986).

Ethics committees need to share their problems and discuss how similar committees work and make decisions. In answer to these needs, several regional networks have been developed across the country, and annual conferences regarding ethics committees are held. A National Ethics Committee Network project was started to provide a solid base of information and materials for committees and to assist them in coordination efforts (Cohen, 1988).

Articles and conferences on ethics committees indicate that while they fill many important functions, problems exist. Committees are generally a volunteer effort with little financial support; seldom do they have secretarial or office support. Additionally, there is some indication that poor leadership and lack of understanding regarding small group process causes committees to become less effective and sometimes inactive (Thornton, 1988).

The problems ethics committees are asked to assist in solving, either in terms of policy making or case consultation, are usually not easy ones. The term ethical dilemma in and of itself indicates controversy. Since one of the purposes of the ethics committee is to open discussion on difficult issues, conflict is a common occurrence.

The problems reported by ethics committees that involve conflict and small group process are several:

1. Many committees, excited about their initial efforts, are thwarted by a lack of communication or leadership. Often these committees remain "paper" committees because attendance dwindles and interest cannot be sustained. Committees need to learn group dynamics techniques including how to run effective meetings, how to help members participate, and how to deal with the interpersonal and role issues between health care disciplines.

2. Committees often report domination by a powerful member, usually a physician. Other members feel frustrated and helpless when this happens since they seldom have the skills to cope with such an issue.

3. Chairs of ethics committees often do not have leadership skills or an understanding of groups.

4. A major criticism of ethics committees is that they get bogged down in what researchers and practitioners of communication refer to as the "group think" syndrome. Decisions are sometimes made that please no one.

5. Committee members do not understand group process.

6. Committee members often do not understand conflict resolution, a necessity when they are dealing with highly charged issues such as euthanasia, abortion and what to do with severely ill newborns.

Corrine Bayley, one of the leaders of the ethics committee movement in the United States is convinced that understanding and implementing successful group process is the key to effective ethics committees. She has spent the last few years educating the many committees for which she is responsible on group process and communication as well as the complicated issues of bioethics. A tough administrator, Bayley talks about "growing an ethics committee," which she likens to an organic process (Bayley, 1986).

As ethics committees begin to understand the need for communication and process consultation, it is difficult for them to know where to turn for assistance. The Society for Bioethics Consultants has been organized to provide guidelines and education to people who consult with committees. It generally consists of persons with legal, medical and philosophical backgrounds. The behavioral science consultant, particularly from the health communication field, is not prominent in the ethics committee milieu.

Health communication experts interested in small group dynamics as well as moral issues could be invaluable to ethics committees and to this group of consultants. Committees often call for help, and health communication experts could make themselves available for such opportunities by calling their local hospitals and volunteering their services as consultants or possibly as ethics committee members.

Ideally, the behavioral scientist or communication specialist who is interested in working with committees should also have an understanding of ethical issues. There are several ways to acquire this expertise. Ethics conferences are held throughout the country. While many of these are three day events, many are more intensive. The Hastings Center in New York and the Kennedy Center in Washington are two leading ethics institutions in the country that sometimes offer courses and other educational experiences. Courses in bioethics are also offered by many universities.

Not only is participation or consultation a possibility, but the opportunities to research ethics committees are rich. In order for committees to function effectively, it would be invaluable to know the answers to the following research questions:

1. How do groups dealing with highly charged topics such as euthanasia, be it active or passive, deal with conflict resolution effectively?

2. How does leadership, both formal and informal, develop in an ethics committee? Who handles task and maintenance roles? Are these roles gender related? How could effective leadership models be designed and implemented?

3. Who plays what role on ethics committees, particularly when the power differential between the doctors and other members of health care is perceived as great?

4. Do ethics committees in different kinds of settings such as hospitals or nursing homes have the same questions, needs, and process and procedural problems?

5. Are ethics committees dealing with problems that could better be dealt with by individuals?

The ethics committee is one of the most interesting health communication settings to develop in some time. It contains the drama of all small groups heightened by the intensity of the health care setting, the importance of dealing with moral issues that impact on all patients and their families, and exciting research opportunities. The field of health communication could make a major contribution to this small group health setting.

Bibliography

Bayley, C. (Oct. 1986) Growing an ethics committee. Conference paper presented at The Ethics Committee Revolution: Coming to terms with substance and process. Eisenhower Medical Center, Rancho Mirage, CA.

Bosford, B. (1986). *Bioethics Committees.* Aspen: Rockville, MD.

Brock, D. (1990) Ethics committees and cost containment. *Hastings Center Report* 29:2:29-33.

Cohen, C. (1988). Birth of a network. *Hastings Center Report* 18, 11-13.

Cranford, R. and Doudera, A. (Eds.) (1984). *Institutional ethics committees and health care decision making.* Ann Arbor, MI.

Hollinger, P. (1989). Hospital ethics committees required by law in Maryland. *Hastings Center Report* 19:1, 23-24.

Macklin, R. (1987) *Mortal Choices.* Boston: Houghton Mifflin Co.

President's Commission for the Study of Ethical Problems in Medicine and Biomedical and Behavioral Research. (1983) *Deciding to forego Life-Sustaining Treatment: Ethical, Medical and Legal Issues in Treatment Decisions.* Washington, DC: U.S. Government Printing Office.

Ross, J. (1986). *Handbook for hospital ethics committees.* American Hospital Association.

Rues, L. and Weaver, B. (1989) Membership issues for hospital ethics committees. *HEC Forum* 1, 127-36.

Siegler, M. (1986) Ethics committees: Decisions by bureaucracy, *Hastings Center Report* 16, 22-24.

Smith, D. (1989) "Case Study Commentary." *Hastings Center Report,* 19(5): 24-25.

Thornton, B. (Oct. 1988) *Future issues for ethics committees.* Paper presented at a conference sponsored by the College of Physicians of Philadelphia, The Hastings Center and the Delaware Valley Ethics Committee Network: Ethics Committees: Moral struggle and strategy in health care institutions. Philadelphia, PA.

Organizational Communication in Health Care

Organizations (such as hospitals, medical centers, nursing homes, clinics, health maintenance organizations, hospices, etc.) are the primary sites for formal health care delivery in the modern health care system. Health care organizations provide both health care services and relevant health information to the public, serving both health care treatment and information dissemination functions. Communication is the primary means by which many different interdependent groups of people that must work together to accomplish health care goals are coordinated within and between complex health care organizations.

Internal organizational communication performs important administrative functions in health care organizations. Communication is directed within health care organizations to coordinate the many complex health care activities of professional staff, clients, and support staff. Formal internal communication is directed up and down the organizational hierarchy and across the many departments of large (often decentralized) health care organizations. For example, downward communication is used by health care administrators to disseminate organizational policies and goals, as well as to provide staff with job directions. Upward communication provides administrators with important feedback from staff at the operational levels of their organizations, helping administrators to make informed decisions about health care policy and practice. Horizontal communication provides representatives of different areas and departments within health care organizations with relevant information for solving commonly encountered problems and coordinating efforts so they are maximizing their energy and resources (promoting synergy).

Informal communication develops within organizations to provide members with information they cannot easily obtain through formal channels. Therefore the more effective formal channels are at disseminating relevant information within organizations, the less need there is for informal channels. However, the less effective the formal channels are at providing members with relevant information, the more informal channels (grapevine) flourish. Kreps and Thornton (1992) recommend that health care administrators work with informal leaders to coordinate formal and informal message systems so the systems overlap and support one another, rather than providing members with contradictory and confusing information. Formal and informal channels of communication do work together in creating organizational cultures and subcultures within health care organizations. These cultures provide members with common interpretations of organizational reality, strongly influencing the norms that guide member behavior in different organizational situations.

External organizational communication is used to coordinate activities between interdependent organizations within the larger health care system. For example, hospitals need to develop effective relationships with public media to encourage media representatives to promote health initiatives and represent their health care services in positive ways, since negative media coverage can undermine public confidence and support for hospitals. Hospitals also use external communication to maintain cooperative relationships with equipment suppliers, educational institutions (that prepare and train health care staff), funding agencies, insurance companies, and accrediting agencies, to name just a few members of the larger health care system. This section of the book examines the multifaceted role of communication in health care organizations, describing how organizational communication can be used to address current administrative challenges in the modern health care system.

The first reading, "Communication in Health Care Organizations," written by Eileen Berlin Ray and Katherine Miller was originally published as a chapter in an edited book on health communication research. This reading takes a strong systems theory perspective of organizations as it reviews current organizational research at multiple hierarchical levels, progressing from interpersonal to group or organizational to interorganizational processes in health care systems. Interestingly, this reading examines the influences of organizational communication in health care on both the consumers of health care and the employees that work within the health care system. After reviewing this reading, you should recognize the complexity of modern health care organizations, the many stresses experienced by consumers and providers of health care, and the importance of social support for all participants within the health care system. This reading is an excellent complement to the article by Ed Roseman in chapter four.

Gary Kreps wrote the second reading in this chapter, entitled "Channelling Information for Organizational Reflexivity," which describes a large-scale organizational development research program in a large urban hospital. The reading describes a hospital that was experiencing very high turnover of nursing staff. Large-scale recruitment of new nurses to staff the hospital was necessary because so many nurses were quitting. Unfortunately, many of the newly recruited nurses also soon left the organization. Kreps describes how research was used to gather relevant information about why the nurses were quitting and to develop a retention program to encourage nurses to stay at their jobs. Recognize as you review this reading that the hospital is viewed as an information system and the retention program is designed to channel relevant information within the organization to improve decision making. Can you describe how this research and development program illustrates the systems theory principle of "requisite variety" (that suggests that the solutions to problems should be as complex as the problems they address)? The hospital's original solution of increasing recruitment to solve nurse turnover clearly violates the principle of requisite variety.

Kreps, G. L. & Thornton, B. C. (1992). *Health Communication: Theory and Practice* 2nd edition. Prospect Heights, IL: Waveland Press.

11

Communication in Health-Care Organizations

By *Eileen Berlin Ray* and
Katherine I. Miller

It is particularly useful to consider the role of communication in health-care organizations from a systems perspective. The input is the patient (and to some extent, his or her family), the throughput is the health care received while the patient is a member of the organization (which may range from aggressive preventive treatment to palliative care), and the output is the result of that care (the patient gets well and leaves the hospital; the patient's final days are made comfortable and dignified; the patient dies but the family feels positive about the care received, etc.). The components within the health-care organization are all the people who have some impact on the care the patient receives. These may include the custodians who keep the facility sanitary, the person who initially interviews the patient when he or she is admitted, orderlies, pharmacists, nurses, doctors, and administrators. Depending on the type of health-care organization, the nature of the task, and other factors, the degree of interdependency among these components will vary. What is critical is that relevant information can be shared quickly and accurately among those who need it. For example, effective communication from a nurse to the pharmacist regarding type and dosage of medication is critical for patient care. If a mistake is made, the patient's life may be jeopardized. The dyadic relationships can also serve a cybernetic function. They may act to amplify or counteract deviations in the health-care process. A doctor may write a prescription order on a patient's chart. The nurse relays that order to the pharmacist. The pharmacist questions the request so the nurse contacts the doctor for clarification. Each dyadic link provides necessary feedback so that the health care system can make adjustments. Thus, a systems framework provides a useful way to think about the role of communication within a health-care organization context.

Reprinted by permission of Lawrence Erlbaum Associates, Inc., Publishers; from E. Berlin Ray and L. Donohew (Eds.), *Communication and Health: Systems and Applications,* pp. 92-107 (1990). Dr. Ray serves on the faculty of the Department of Communication at Cleveland State University and Dr. Miller serves on the faculty of the Department of Communication at Arizona State University.

Within this framework, it is necessary to consider both the internal and external communication processes and their impact on health-care delivery. To understand the potential effects of the organization/patient and intraorganizational interdependencies, we distinguish between viewing the health-care organization as (a) a *dispenser* of care and, (b) a *cause* of health-care needs for the providers. As a dispenser, the focus is on how the dynamics within the organization enable the health-care providers to meet the needs of its patients in the best possible way. Thus, we can look at communication processes within the organization as they affect patient care. The interface of the providers with the patients, their families, and the community are of particular relevance here. As a cause of health-care needs, the focus shifts from patient care to how the stresses of providing health care influence the health of the providers. Of particular importance here are the stress levels of health-care providers and the negative physical and emotional/mental effects of dysfunctional stress. As Dye (1985) noted, "It is ironic that an organization dedicated to restoring health and promoting well-being often is detrimental to the health and well-being of the people working there" (p. 3).

Obviously, the relationship between the organization as dispenser and as cause is one of interdependence. If the provider's health needs (both physical and emotional) are not met, the quality of patient care will suffer. And if the organization structure is such that providers feel their ability to provide quality care is impeded, their health/attitudes will be negatively affected.

For the organizational purposes of this chapter, our examination of communication in health-care organizations focuses first on the organization as the dispenser of health care and second on the provision of health care as a source of stress for employees of health-care organizations. Both of these issues are considered by examining communication within the organizational context at the interpersonal, work group, organization, and interorganizational levels.

The Organization as Dispenser

The goal of any health-care organization, from emergency treatment centers to traditional hospitals, is to provide quality care to its patients. What is considered quality care can be ascertained in a number of ways from a number of perspectives. For physicians, it may be the number of remissions or successful treatments of patients. For nurses, it may be the feeling that they provided care that improved the quality of their patients' lives. For patients and their families, quality includes all of the aforementioned as well as positive interpersonal relationships with the caregivers. Patients who like their health-care providers, feel that they are listened to, are treated kindly, and generally perceive the interpersonal dynamics as positive, tend to be more satisfied with their medical care (Burgoon et al., 1987; Kreps & Thornton, 1984; Pendleton & Hasler,

1983; Street & Wiemann, 1987). Families, typically not competent in the technical aspects of the treatment their family member is receiving, base their impressions on how they are treated by the staff they encounter. They make attributions of good health care if they are shown consideration whenever they are in the health-care setting (Nyquist, Booms, & Hasler, 1989). In addition, patients and families who feel a positive relationship with their health-care providers may be less likely to take legal action against a health-care provider (May, 1985). So although the actual technical care that is dispensed is obviously critical, the relational components of how it is dispensed are also of great importance.

Health-care organizations differ from other types of organizations in many ways. Of particular importance is the nature of the organizational task. Whether it is physical, mental, or a combination health-care facility, the urgency, often life and death, of patient and family needs is great (Thompson, 1986). The information exchange between health-care professionals is critical to ensure quality care for patients and it is the coordination of all relevant people and activities that is essential for successful health-care delivery (Kreps, 1988). It is useful to examine how communication provides this coordination in health-care organizations at the interpersonal, group, organizational structure, and interorganizational levels. A discussion of each follows.

Interpersonal Level

Within the health-care organization, communication at the interpersonal, or dyadic level, may occur between the health-care provider and patient, between two health-care providers (i.e., doctor-nurse, nurse-nurse), or between provider and technician. Expanding the system boundaries to the organizational context, however, changes the interdependencies and dynamics of these dyadic relationships. If we conceptualize patient care within a health-care organization as a series of dyadic linkages, a break in any of the links affects the quality of patient care. For example, data collected in the initial patient interview is used to make critical decisions regarding patient care (Barsky et al., 1980; Thompson, 1986). The patient interview has been described as a special type of two-way communication (Mason & Swash, 1975). If the interviewer is not properly trained in question asking as well as interpreting subtle nonverbal cues of the patient, the resulting information will be incomplete or biased and the resulting health care will be less than optimal.

It is this transactional nature of the communication process between the provider and recipient that can act in a deviation counteracting or amplifying manner. The degree of coordination between the physician and patient is critical for effective health care (Helman, 1985; Mathews, 1983) and may be influenced by the mutual information exchange between the doctor and patient (Argyle, 1983; Lucas, 1985). Feedback is critical for this function to be served.

Unfortunately, many times this does not occur. Patients may be unable or unwilling to adequately communicate their medical concerns to the doctor (Friedman & DiMatteo, 1979) and physicians may not probe subtle verbal or nonverbal cues of the patient.

Within the organizational context, the dyadic linkages, beginning with the patient interview and extending to the ties that are enacted to care for that patient, can only be successful to the extent that the information gathered and shared at each linkage point is accurate. Feedback at each point is critical to provide the necessary counteracting or amplifying functions. Effective information gathering and exchange is also essential. However, each additional link in the communication chain increases the system's interdependence and opportunity for distortion. Thus, the more dyadic links involved in the patient's care within the organizational context, the greater the chance that some degree of communication breakdown will occur and ultimately affect the patient's care.

Work-Group Level

Expanding the system boundaries to examine group communication within the organizational context results in greater interdependencies among team members and requires greater coordination and control of communication and activities (Farace, Monge, & Russell, 1977). One example of groups within the organizational context is health-care teams. Health-care teams are particularly prevalent in the care for the terminally ill. These teams are multidisciplinary and typically include a primary physician, a nurse, social workers, patient-care coordinator, an administrator, and the patient or family (Blues & Zerwekh, 1984). Ideally, the health-care team should work in concert and draw on the diverse expertise of its members. The team should serve the necessary deviation amplifying or counteracting function, keeping the system in a state of dynamic homeostasis in meeting the health-care needs of the patient. In this way, changes can be made in the health care provided while maintaining the necessary balance among the team members. However, it is often the team members, as well as the organizational context, that exacerbate, rather than ameliorate, problems (Vachon, 1987).

In addition, health-care teams are expected to work together, ignoring real or imagined differences and egos, for altruistic goals. However, years of academic training, social and cultural factors, and perceptions of statuses assigned to the health-care professions cannot be ignored. In addition, most have been trained to work independently, not interdependently. They often become team members with no advanced communication training or skills in group dynamics and find it difficult to cross traditional professional (Mount & Voyer, 1980) or gender hierarchies (Campbell-Heider & Pollock, 1987). As Mount and Voyer (1980), quoting Rubin, noted:

> It is naive to bring together a highly diverse group of people and expect
> that, by calling them a team, they will in fact behave as a team. It is ironic
> indeed to realize that a football team spends 40 hours a week practicing
> teamwork for the two hours on Sunday afternoon when their team really
> counts. Teams in organizations seldom spend two hours per year practicing
> when their ability to function as a team counts 40 hours per week. (p. 466)

In addition to health-care teams, it is critical that work-group members are able to coordinate their activities in a timely fashion within the health-care organization. However, this is often difficult to do. In a study by Ray (1983a), hospital nurses reported several stressors inherent in the organizational context. These included not being treated like a professional, the politics of the hospital, inadequate information from doctors about patients, and dealing with inefficient departments. Conflict with physicians (Gray-Toft, 1980; Vachon, Lyall, & Freeman, 1978) as well as support staff and administration (Yancik, 1984) and limitations of the physical facility (Ray, Nichols, & Perritt, 1987) are also likely to upset the necessary balance among work group members.

Organizational Level

The structure of a health-care organization has a significant impact on its ability to coordinate activities effectively and subsequently dispense adequate health care. It is both the interconnectedness among different aspects of work tasks and the interdependence among units that are critical (Charns & Schaefer, 1983). This interconnectedness and interdependence can only be accomplished through communication (Costello & Pettegrew, 1979; Kreps, 1986).

Several characteristics lead to effective and efficient coordination among interconnected tasks. Coordination must be increased to the extent that the organization's structure separates components of the work that are highly interconnected. This need for coordination is influenced by factors such as task uncertainty, size and interdependence, and influence (Charns & Schaefer, 1983). For example, the greater the task uncertainty, the greater the need for coordination. When uncertainty is low, departments can act in a routine way, with little need for additional coordination. However, when uncertainty is high, coordination becomes critical. A patient suffering from a rare disease or whose condition is quickly deteriorating for no obvious medical reason increases uncertainty and the need for coordination and information exchange among those caring for the patient (Kreps, 1988).

The larger the organization, the greater the need for coordination. The more departments involved in providing the health care, the more complex the coordination becomes. Increases in the number of links in the communication chain result in more complicated control and coordination processes. As Farace et al. (1977) observed, "If messages must pass through the hands of many people for a critical act of coordination, they may become distorted and the coordination effort may fail. If control messages must be broadcast to many individuals in a short time period, no communication mechanism may exist which can do the job" (p. 16).

Interdependence refers to the necessary interrelationships among work units (Charns & Schaefer, 1983). The most common, complex, and difficult to coordinate in health-care organizations is reciprocal interdependence (Thompson, 1967). This occurs when both units affect each other. For example, all of the units involved in the care of a patient are reciprocally interdependent.

Reciprocal interdependence requires both formal and informal communication networks to maximize information exchange and reduce information equivocality. Both of these networks require the support of the organizational administration and the various units. Reciprocal interdependence can best be conceptualized as reciprocal communication linkages within these networks. This reciprocity can help ensure the accurate and timely exchange of information among these linkages that is critical for successful health care delivery.

Interorganizational Level

At the interorganizational level, coordination among the components of an integrated health-care system becomes particularly crucial. As health-care provision is viewed as a community problem, the ways in which a wide range of health-care organizations can coordinate their efforts will determine the quality of care available to patients. For example, a number of national programs have been instituted to develop community-based systems of health-care provision in which hospitals, medical schools, public health agencies, and home health-care providers attempt to work together in a cohesive program of health education, prevention, and treatment. Thus, understanding the ways communication works to link these interorganizational efforts is essential to effective coordination and health-care provision.

Eisenberg et al. (1985) recently reviewed theory and research on communication linkages in interorganizational systems. As a great deal of the research they reviewed considered health-care organizations (see, e.g., White & Vlasak, 1970), Eisenberg et al.'s taxonomy of interorganizational communication is particularly relevant in the health-care context. They proposed that interorganizational links can involve either information (i.e., symbolic) exchange or material exchange (i.e., the flow of money, goods, and personnel). Both types of exchange are crucial for the most effective interorganizational linkages. For example, an effective community-based cancer control program would require health-care organizations to exchange information about specific patients and specific programs, as well as exchange personnel for training and a wide variety of material necessary for the effective provision of education and treatment. Eisenberg et al. further proposed that interorganizational linkages can involve a personal link (e.g., between physicians from separate hospitals who share information over dinner or at the golf course), a representative link (e.g., between officials at a county health agency and a medical school attempting to coordinate health education efforts in the community), or an institutional link (a link between two organizations that does not specifically involve individuals). Again, the literature clearly suggests that all three of these kinds of links are necessary for effective coordination among organizations. Eisenberg et al. (1985), however, suggested that forging such links can be difficult, particularly among professionals in health-care organizations. As they noted:

> Perceived status distinctions between different kinds of professionals (notably physicians and social service professionals) limit the extent to which personal linkages are formed between members of these two groups (Monge, Farace, Miller, & Eisenberg, 1983). For representative linkages between individuals, the high turnover associated with professionals can impact negatively on the stability of interorganizational systems, since the turnover of key liaison or boundary role occupants can interrupt long-standing patterns of formal and informal information exchange. Particularly in interorganizational networks where linkages are voluntary, personal, and information-oriented, exchange relations which have developed over time are vulnerable to the effects of professional turnover (pp. 250-251).

The Organization as Cause

It is clear at this point that the nature of communication within health-care organizations has a significant impact on the quality of care received by patients. The literature just reviewed suggests that quality care depends on effective communication within a wide range of interpersonal linkages, effective communication within the work group, and coordination among organizational subsystems and between health-care organizations within a community. Our attention thus far, however, has centered on the effects of communication on the care provided by health-care professionals. The other side of the coin should be considered as well. That is, communication within health-care organizations can have an important impact on the individuals providing the care (i.e., doctors, nurses, administrators, social workers). Most of the literature in this area has considered how the provision of health care can be stressful to individuals and the extent to which health-care professionals are prone to the syndrome that has come to be known as burnout. The remainder of this chapter considers how communication within health-care organizations can affect the level of stress and burnout experienced by workers within these organizations. Once again, we consider several system levels within these organizations, although we should remember that these levels are necessarily interdependent on each other.

Interpersonal Level

Burnout has been defined as a wearing down from the chronic emotional pressures of human service work (Pines, Aronson, & Kafry, 1981) and is characterized by physical, emotional, and mental exhaustion (Maslach, 1982; Pines et al., 1981), by a decreasing sense of personal accomplishment (Maslach, 1982), and by a tendency to depersonalize care recipients (Maslach, 1982). The provision of health care almost always requires the establishment of interpersonal relationships between the health-care provider and the recipient. Maslach (1982) has suggested that this interpersonal relationship is the major cause of burnout among all human service workers, health-care professionals included. As she noted, "what is unique about burnout is that the stress arises from the social interaction between helper and recipient" (p. 3).

Pines (1982) suggested that the interpersonal relationships between a health-care provider and recipient are unusual in that the care provider always gives — and rarely receives — emotional resources. This relational asymmetry places a great deal of pressure on the care provider to be communicatively competent, and this pressure can ultimately lead to burnout. Thus, it would seem reasonable to suggest that the nature of the interpersonal communication between the health-care provider and care recipient could influence the extent to which the care provider experiences negative outcomes. Lief and Fox (1963) coined the term "detached concern" to describe a necessary condition for medical students in providing quality care. They suggested that avoiding burnout requires health-care providers to feel a true concern for the patient while at the same time maintaining a large share of emotional distance. Miller, Stiff, and Ellis (1988) supported this notion, finding that caregivers in a psychiatric hospital who perceived themselves as most communicatively responsive were those who had high levels of empathic concern for patients but low levels of emotional contagion. Perceived communicative responsiveness, in turn, had a strong effect on the level of burnout experienced by care providers.

Of course, the relationship between caregiver and care recipient is only one of the many interpersonal relationships within a health-care organization. Relationships among caregivers can also have a large impact on the well-being of employees. For example, Marshall (1980) reviewed literature highlighting relationships with doctors as a potential source of stress for many nurses. She noted that "the traditional role segregation between the responsible diagnosing and treating doctor and the caring nurse is not easily maintained even if both parties agree with its underlying justice" (p. 32). Relationships with family members can also be stressful to caregivers in that "they represent a third party with their own separate attribution of meanings, reactions, and needs for support" (Marshall, 1980, p. 31). Perhaps the most important single relationship beyond the caregiver-care recipient relationship, however, is between the caregiver and his or her supervisor.

A number of writers have pointed to the importance of support from the supervisor in reducing job stress and burnout, particularly in caregiving organizations (see Ray, 1987, for a review of this literature). The communicative support of a supervisor can be useful in a number of ways. First, a supportive supervisor can serve to reduce the level of ambiguity a health-care professional feels about his or her role. Informational support of this kind — particularly providing workers with an opportunity to participate in the decision-making process — is crucial, for role ambiguity has been found to be a major contributor to stress and burnout in workers in general (Kahn, 1978) and in health professionals in particular (Miller, Ellis, Zook, & Lyles, 1988). A supportive supervisor can also provide emotional support by allowing the care provider to vent feelings and by letting the stressed worker know that he or she is not alone. Marshall (1980) suggested that staff meetings — in addition to providing informational support — can supply needed emotional support. "Nurses should have the opportunity to express and share their reactions to their work in regular staff meetings and . . . training should be given to help them understand and cope with anxiety about death and dying" (p. 53).

Work-Group Level

The work group within a health-care organization can serve both as a source of stress and as an important coping mechanism for individuals suffering from stress and burnout. Support from coworkers has long been noted as an important buffer against workplace stressors. It is assumed that coworkers are in an optimal position to provide support, as they have the greatest understanding of the workplace and its inherent stressors (House, 1981; Ray, 1987). Especially in health-care organizations, friends and families may not have sufficient understanding of the workplace context to provide the emotional and informational support necessary for effective coping. However, communication with coworkers can be a double-edged sword. Adelman's (1986) investigation of the "contagion effect" among nurses suggests that the same communication behavior that can serve the useful purpose of venting and sharing frustrations can also lead health-care providers to higher levels of stress as they vicariously experience the stresses of their coworkers as well.

Research supports the importance of work-group linkages as both a positive and negative factor in the lives of health-care employees. A survey of 1,000 nurses (Steffen, 1980) found that although relationships within the work group were the second greatest source of satisfaction at work ("being part of a skilled team" and "peer recognition and support," p. 46), these relationships were also the second greatest source of stress: problems with other nurses ("the continuously competitive atmosphere, along with the lack of comraderie," p. 51) and problems with physicians and supervisors. Likewise, Ray (1983a) found interpersonal relationships between nurses and others in a hospital to be highly stressful. However, Nievaard (1987) found that improved communication among nurses in a Dutch hospital did not significantly affect their attitudes toward patients. Rather, it was problems with the doctors and hospital administration that were positively related to negative attitudes toward patients.

Organizational Level

At the organizational level, the structure of ties among health-care providers appears to affect their ability to cope with the stress inherent in their job and buffer ill health. It is these resulting networks that can impede or enhance the amount of support perceived by providers.

Support is inherently communicative in nature. According to Albrecht and Adelman (1984), support is "the way in which communication behaviors tie an individual to his or her social environment and functions to enable the individual to positively relate to that environment" (p. 4). The communication of support within health-care organizations is developed and maintained through the ongoing, regular interactions among its members (Wellman, 1981). The degree of availability and accessibility of support largely results from the structure of ties organization members have with each other (Gottlieb, 1981). As noted by House (1981), "Flows of social support occur primarily in the context of relatively stable social relationships rather than fleeting interactions among strangers" (p. 29). Of particular importance is the health-care provider's location in the informal communication network as a mediator of negative health outcomes. For example, Anderson and Gray-Toft (1982) found nurses on the day shift with high stress and burnout were located in the center of the support network, whereas evening and night-shift nurses were not. Ray (1983b) found that nurses in a children's hospital who were integrated in their work unit reported less burnout but no less stress than those less integrated. These findings were replicated by Dye (1985) with a sample of intensive care hospital nurses.

However, it is important to recognize that these network ties may act to increase, rather than decrease, stress and burnout. If the content of the ongoing communication is negative, interaction may act in a deviation amplifying manner, increasing the provider's negative affect. This has been referred to as the "contagion effect" (Adelman, 1986; Cherniss, 1980; Ray, 1983b) or reverse buffering (Beehr, 1985). The resulting stress and burnout then must be counteracted with positively valenced messages, often introduced through formal organizational-level interventions (Edelwich, 1980). In addition to message content, research in nonhealth related organizations suggests that network characteristics such as the degree of reciprocity, multiplexity, and strength of communication ties are also negatively related to stress and burnout (Ray, 1986).

Interorganizational Level

The importance of links between organizations for the effective delivery of coordinated health care was discussed earlier. In establishing these interorganizational linkages, and in dealing with the consumers of health care, many health providers find themselves on the "edges" of organizations. Although they are officially affiliated with a particular hospital, office, or health agency, a majority of these individuals' time is spent interacting with outsiders such as patients, families, representatives of other health-care organizations, and government and regulatory agency officials. Clearly, as noted earlier, the quality of these extra-organizational linkages will impact the extent to which it is possible to deliver high quality care. In addition, however, the very process of spanning organizational boundaries can cause extensive stress for the individual employee or health-care provider.

The term *boundary spanner* was coined by Adams (1980) to describe an organizational role in which an individual serves in some way to functionally relate an organization to its environment. Adams noted a number of boundary activities these individuals engage in: (a) transacting organizational inputs and outputs, (b) filtering inputs and outputs, (c) searching for and collecting information, (d) representing the organization, and (e) buffering the organization from external threats. In a health-care organization, boundary-spanning activities would include a wide range of contact with patients and families, supply procurement, establishing and maintaining contacts with other health-care organizations, dealing with insurance agencies, and so on. In short, the very nature of a health-care organization requires extensive boundary spanning activities by a wide range of organizational employees.

Boundary-spanning activities can often be stressful for organizational employees. Adams (1976,1980) noted that buffering an organization can lead to role conflict, stress, and tension for the boundary spanner in several ways. First, the boundary spanner can experience tension from trying to balance the needs of the organization with the needs of the "outsiders" with whom transactions are taking place. This stress is particularly crucial for individuals in public relations roles, for Adams (1980) noted that "giving the impression to outsiders that their voice is being heard and given weight conflicts with the ethical principle that one should be truthful" (p. 350). Adams (1980) also noted a second source of stress for the boundary spanner: "the frequent hostility of outsiders, especially members of 'activist' groups, attempting to induce change in the organization" (p. 350).

More specific to the health-care context, however, is the specific boundary-spanning activity of contact with patients and their families. Literature on caregivers has repeatedly noted the detrimental effects of large caseloads on the psychological and physical health of human service personnel (Daley, 1979; Maslach & Pines, 1977; Pines & Maslach, 1978). These researchers note that constant interaction with individuals in need of help can be extremely stressful, especially when there is little positive feedback received from the care recipient and when there seems little hope that the level of contact will be reduced. This problem is particularly acute in chronically understaffed health fields such as nursing (Jacobson & McGrath, 1983).

Summary

We noted at the beginning that the systems perspective was particularly crucial for a consideration of communication in health-care organizations. The issues we have reviewed clarify this point by highlighting the crucial interdependence among health-care providers in a variety of organizational roles, their patients and the patients' families, and the larger community environment in which the health-care organization exists. Clearly, providing quality health care requires coordination at all levels of the organizational system — coordination between the health-care provider and recipient, coordination among health-care team members, coordination among disparate departments within the health-care organizations, and interorganizational coordination among community agencies. This coordinated effort can pay high dividends in terms of the quality of care received by the patient. Unfortunately, the provision of care can also mean high costs for the professional health-care provider in terms of the stress and burnout associated with the caregiving role, although clear role definitions and social support from within the organization can serve to lessen this risk. It is only through an increased understanding of the interdependence of health-care providers and their patients within the health-care organization that we can improve the quality of life for both the caregiver and the care recipient.

References

Adams, J. S. 1976. The structure and dynamics of behavior in organization boundary roles. In M. D. Dunnette (ed.), *Handbook of industrial and organizational psychology* (pp. 1175-99). Chicago: Rand McNally.

Adams, J. S. 1980. Interorganizational processes and organization boundary activities. *Research in Organizational Behavior*, 2, 321-55.

Adelman, M. B. 1986. The contagion effect: A study on stress and the provision of support. Unpublished doctoral dissertation, University of Washington, Seattle, WA.

Albrecht, T. L., & Adelman, M. B. 1984. Social support and life stress: New directions for communication research. *Human Communication Research*, 11, 3-32.

Anderson, J. G. & Gray-Toft, P. A. 1982. *Stress, burnout, and turnover among health professionals: A social network approach*. Paper presented at the annual meeting of the International Sociological Association, Mexico City.

Argyle, M. 1983. Doctor-patient skills. In D. Pendleton & J. Hasler (eds.), *Doctor-patient communication* (pp. 57-74). London: Academic Press.

Barsky, A. J., Kazis, L. E., Freiden, R. B., Goroll, A. H., Hatem, C. J., & Lawrence, R. S. 1980. Evaluating the interview in primary care medicine. *Social Science and Medicine*, 14A, 653.

Beehr, T. A. 1985. The role of social support in coping with organizational stress. In T. A. Beehr & R. S. Bhagat (eds.), *Human stress and cognition in organizations: An integrated perspective* (pp. 375-98). New York: Wiley.

Blues, A. G., & Zerwekh, J. V. 1984. *Hospice and palliative nursing care*. Orlando, FL: Grune & Stratton.

Burgoon, J. K., Pfau, M., Parrott, R., Birk, T., Coker, R., & Burgoon, M. 1987. Relational communication, satisfaction, compliance-gaining strategies, and compliance in communication between physicians and patients. *Communication Monographs*, 54, 307-24.

Campbell-Heider, N., & Pollock, D. 1987. Barriers to physician-nurse collegiality: An anthropological perspective. *Social Science and Medicine*, 25(5), 421-25.

Charns, M. P., & Schaefer, M. J. 1983. *Health care organizations*. Englewood Cliffs, NJ: Prentice-Hall.

Cherniss, C. 1980. *Staff burnout: Job stress in the social services*. Beverly Hills, CA: Sage.

Costello, D., & Pettegrew, L. 1979. Health communication theory and research: An overview of health organizations. In D. Nimmo (ed.), *Communication yearbook* 3 (pp. 607-23). New Brunswick, NJ: Transaction-International Communication Association.

Daley, M. R. 1979. Preventing worker burnout in child welfare. *Child Welfare*, 58, 443-50.

Dye, F. W. 1985. *Supportive communication networks and job stress: A study of intensive care nurses*. Unpublished master's thesis, University of Kentucky, Lexington, KY.

Edelwich, J. 1980. *Burn-out: Stages of disillusionment in the helping professions*. New York: Human Sciences Press.

Eisenberg, E. M., Farace, R. V., Monge, P. R., Bettinghaus, E. P., Kurchner-Hawkins, R., Miller, K. I., & White, L. L. 1985. Communication linkages in interorganizational systems: Review and synthesis. In B. Dervin & M. J. Voigt (eds.), *Advances in communication science* (Vol. 6, pp. 231-61). Norwood, NJ: Ablex.

Farace, R. V., Monge, P. R., & Russell, H. 1977. *Communicating and organizing*. Reading, MA: Addison-Wesley.

Friedman, H. S., & DiMatteo, M. R. 1979. *Health care as an interpersonal process*. *Journal of Social Issues*, 35, 82-89.

Gottlieb, B. H. 1981. Social networks and social support in community health. In B. H. Gottlieb (ed.), *Social networks and social support* (pp. 11-42). Beverly Hills CA: Sage.

Gray-Toft, P. 1980. Effectiveness of a counseling support program for hospice nurses. *Journal of Counseling Psychology*, 27(4), 346-54.

Helman, C. G. 1985. Communication in primary care: The role of patient and practitioner explanatory models. *Social Science and Medicine*, 20(9), 923-31.

House, J. S. 1981. *Work stress and social support*. Reading, MA: Addison-Wesley.

Jacobson, S. F., & McGrath, H. M. (eds.). 1983. *Nurses under stress*. New York: Wiley.

Kahn, R. 1978. Job burnout: Prevention and remedies. *Public Welfare*, 36(2), 61-63.

Kreps, G. 1988. The pervasive role of information in health and health care: Implications for health communication policy. In J. Anderson (ed.), *Communication yearbook* 11 (pp. 238-276). Menlo Park, CA: Sage.

Kreps, G. 1986. *Organizational communication: Theory and practice*. White Plains, NY: Longman.

Kreps, G., & Thornton, B. 1984. *Health communication*. New York: Longman.

Lief, H. I., & Fox, R. C. 1963. Training for "detached concern" in medical students. In H. I. Lief, V. F. Lief, & N. R. Lief (eds.), *The psychological basis of medical practice* (pp. 12-35). New York: Harper & Row.

Lucas, I. R. 1985, August. *The effects of initial interaction on uncertainty, rapport, and interpersonal attraction*. Paper presented at the Summer Conference on Health Communication, Evanston, IL.

Marshall, J. 1980. Stress amongst nurses. In C. L. Cooper & J. Marshall (eds.), *White collar and professional stress* (pp. 19-59). New York: Wiley.

Maslach, C. 1982. *Burnout: The cost of caring*. Englewood Cliffs, NJ: Prentice-Hall.

Maslach, C., & Pines, A. 1977. The burn-out syndrome in the day care setting. *Child Care Quarterly*, 6, 100-13.

Mason, S., & Swash, M. 1975. *Hutchinson's clinical methods* (17th ed.). London: Bailliere Tindall.

Mathews, J. J. 1983. The communication process in clinical settings. *Social Science and Medicine*, 17, 1371.

May, M. L. 1985, August. *Patients and doctors in conflict: The nature of patients' complaints and what they do about them*. Paper presented at the Summer Conference on Health Communication, Evanston, IL.

Miller, K. I., Ellis, B. H., Zook, E. G., & Lyles, J. S. 1988. *An integrated model of communication, stress, and burnout in the workplace*. Unpublished manuscript, Department of Communication, Michigan State University, East Lansing.

Miller, K. I., Stiff, J. B., & Ellis, B. H. 1988. Communication and empathy as precursors to burnout among human service workers. *Communication Monographs*, 55, 250-65.

Monge, P. R., Farace, R. V., Miller, K. I., & Eisenberg, E. M. 1983, May. *Life cycle changes in interorganizational information networks*. Paper presented at the annual convention of the International Communication Association, Dallas, TX.

Mount, B., & Voyer, J. 1980. Staff stress in palliative/hospice care. In I. Ajemian & B. Mount (eds.), *The RVH manual on palliative/hospice care* (pp. 457-88). New York: The Free Press.

Nievaard, A. C. 1987. Communication climate and patient care: Causes and effects of nurses' attitudes to patients. *Social Science and Medicine*, 24(9), 777-84.

Nyquist, J. D., Booms, B. H., & Hasler, J. 1989. *Communication behaviors for enhancing family and resident satisfaction in nursing homes*. Paper presented at the annual meeting of the Western Speech Communication Association, Spokane, WA.

Pendleton, D., & Hasler, J. 1983. *Doctor-patient communication*. London: Academic Press.

Pines, A. M. 1982. Helpers' motivation and the burnout syndrome. In T. A. Wills (ed.), *Basic processes in helping relationships* (pp. 453-75). New York: Academic Press.

Pines, A.M., Aronson, E., & Kafry, D. 1981. *Burnout: From tedium to personal growth*. New York: The Free Press.

Pines, A. M., & Maslach. C. 1978. Characteristics of staff burnout in mental health settings. *Hospital and Community Psychiatry*, 29, 233-37.

Ray, E. B. 1987. Support relationships and occupational stress in the workplace. In T. L. Albrecht, M. B. Adelman, & Associates, (eds.), *Communicating social support* (pp. 172-91). Newbury Park, CA: Sage.

Ray, E. B. 1986. *Communication network roles as mediators of job stress and burnout: Case studies of two organizations.* Paper presented at the annual meeting of the Speech Communication Association, Chicago, IL.

Ray, E. B. 1983a. Identifying job stress in a human service organization. *Journal of Applied Communication Research*, 11, 109-19.

Ray, E. B. 1983b. Job burnout from a communication perspective. In R. N. Bostrom (ed.), *Communication yearbook 7* (pp. 738-55). Beverly Hills, CA: Sage.

Ray, E. B., Nichols, M. R., & Perritt, L. J. 1987. A model of job stress and burnout. *The Hospice Journal*, 3(2/3), 3-28.

Steffen, S. 1980. Perceptions of stress: 1800 nurses tell their stories. In K. Claus & J. Bailey (eds.), *Living with stress and promoting well-being* (pp. 38-58). St. Louis: C. V. Mosby.

Street, R. L., Jr., & Wiemann, J. M. 1987. Patient satisfaction with physicians' interpersonal involvement, expressiveness, and dominance. In M. McLaughlin (ed.), *Communication yearbook* 10 (pp. 591-612). Newbury Park, CA: Sage.

Thompson, J. D. 1967. *Organizations in action.* New York: McGraw-Hill.

Thompson, T. L. 1986. *Communication for health professionals.* New York: Harper & Row.

Vachon, M. L. S. 1987. Team stress in palliative/hospice care. *The Hospice Journal*, 3(2/3), 75-103.

Vachon, M. L. S., Lyall, W. A. L., & Freeman, S. J. J. 1978. Measurement and management of stress in health professionals working with advanced cancer patients. *Death Education*, 1, 365-75.

Wellman, B. 1981. Applying network analysis to the study of support. In B. H. Gottlieb (ed.), *Social networks and social support* (pp. 171-200). Beverly Hills, CA: Sage.

White, P. E., & Vlasak, G. J. (eds.). 1970. *Interorganizational research in health.* Baltimore, MD: Department of Behavioral Sciences, Johns Hopkins University.

Yancik, R. 1984. Coping with hospice work stress. *Journal of Psycho-social Oncology*, 2(2), 19-35.

12

Channelling Information for Organizational Reflexivity

A Field Research and Development Study of Nurse Turnover and Retention in a Large Urban Health Care Organization

By Gary L. Kreps

Organizations, like human beings, must be able to adapt to survive (French, Bell, & Zawacki, 1978; Lippitt, 1977). Effective organizational development efforts begin with gathering information about organizational performance gaps to determine which aspects of the organization need to be improved to promote successful adaptation (Knight and McDaniel, 1979; Kreps, 1986; Rogers & Agarwala-Rogers, 1978). Important sources of such information are organization members who can often provide operational information about specific problems they face that hinder the performance of organizational activities.

In this study nurses were identified as important sources of relevant operational information in a large urban public hospital (Salem & Williams, 1984). The phenomenon of high turnover of nursing staff was examined by gathering information from nurses about the specific problems they face that may lead them to terminate their employment with the hospital and translating these data into a nurse retention organizational development program. The data gathered were utilized to develop organization-specific intervention strategies and organizational improvements in the hospital. Implementation of formal feedback channels between nursing staff and hospital administration served to provide nurses with organizationally approved communication channels for expressing their dissatisfactions about the hospital. Feedback loops were designed to help the hospital administration make informed decisions, based upon the expertise of nursing staff, to direct the development and introduction

This article was originally presented at the annual convention of the International Communication Association in Chicago (May, 1986).

Funding for this study was supplied from grants by Wishard Memorial Hospital of Indianapolis, Indiana. The following individuals assisted in collecting data for this study: Helene Cross, Jeff Golc, and Jim L. Query, Jr.

of organizational innovations needed to increase retention of nuring staff. The retention organizational development program was designed primarily to increase retention of nursing staff and also to help the hospital administration become more aware of operational problems, increase reflexiveness of the health care organization, and direct the resolution of problems (Kreps, 1986).

The Organizational Costs of Nurse Turnover and Recruitment

High turnover rates of nursing staff in hospitals across the nation have caused many problems (Filoromo & Ziff, 1980; Wandelt, Pierce, & Widdowson, 1981; Wolf, 1981). Excessive employee turnover has been linked to several organizational problems including increased costs (recruiting, hiring, assimilation, training, replacement, out-processing), disruption of social and communication structures, productivity loss, loss of high performers, decreased satisfaction among stayers, increase of undifferentiated turnover control strategies, and negative public relations from those who leave (Mobley, 1982; 1977). High nurse turnover can frustrate remaining organization members and lead to disruption of work flow, increased workload during and immediately after search for replacement, decreased cohesion, and decreased commitment — in addition to the loss of functionally-valued coworkers (Mobley, 1982).

Nurses who leave hospitals take with them valuable information about how to get things done in their organizations, something referred to as "organizational intelligence" (Kreps, 1986; Weick, 1979). Hospitals lose even more organizational intelligence when nurses are taken off their jobs to train newly recruited nurses. Newly recruited nurses often fill jobs that are difficult for them to accomplish because they do not have the organizational skills that come with experience (Kreps & Thornton, 1984). Mistakes made by newly recruited nurses can make the work life of other hospital nurses frustrating, decrease their job satisfaction, and lead to increased turnover.

The administrative philosophy behind the retention organizational development program was a radical departure from traditional recruitment responses to nurse turnover. The recruitment approach views nurses as cogs in the hospital machine that can be replaced. Accordingly, as nurse turnover increases, hospitals seek new nurses to replace those who leave. The retention program rejected this philosophy and suggested hospitals should devote more energy to keeping nurses satisfied and productive than to replacing nurses. The retention philosophy argued that the more a hospital replaces nurses, the more problems are created for the organization through loss of organizational intelligence. Reacting to nurse turnover by replacing nurses does not help solve the problems underlying turnover and, in fact, may exacerbate those underlying organizational problems.

Identification of Relevant Performance Gaps

A field-study investigating nurses' evaluations of organizational climate and job satisfaction/dissatisfaction was conducted to identify problems causing operational difficulties at a large urban public hospital in the Midwest. At the initiation of the study, the hospital was experiencing a high rate of nurse turnover, approximately 35% annually. The study attempted to identify the primary reasons for turnover and to use that information to develop procedures for nurse retention and organizational development.

Three concurrent research phases were used as assessment tools in this study to identify the primary issues underlying nurse turnover: questionnaires, in-depth interviews, and focus-group discussions. These three research phases combined quantitative and qualitative methods of analysis, providing a means of "method triangulation" to interpret organizational reality through the eyes of organization members (Albrecht & Ropp, 1982; Jick, 1979). The questionnaires were used to identify general issues of concern to nursing staff members, while the interviews and the focus groups were used to provide in-depth analysis and recommendations for relieving problems that were identified. The questionnaire was used to examine hospital communication climate and nurse job satisfaction. The climate scale was adapted from the "Mental Health Center Climate Questionnaire" developed and validated by Hunter (1976; 1978). There are three dimensions to the climate scale: administrative recognition, staff congruence, and facility conditions. Nurse job satisfaction was measured with the "Job Descriptive Index" developed and validated by Smith, Kendall, and Hulin (1969). There are five dimensions to the job satisfaction scale: work, supervision, pay, promotions, and coworkers. The questionnaire was made available to the total population of nurses (n = 535) at their work locations.

The in-depth, open-ended interviews were conducted with a selective sample (n = 49) of nurses who were identified as "key communicators" (knowledgeable and active members of the hospital's organizational culture) by administrators and staff nurses. The interviews checked and expanded upon the primary issues concerning climate and job satisfaction identified in the questionnaire, asking respondents to evaluate their work lives, identify specific areas of work satisfaction and dissatisfaction, and suggest areas for potential improvement within the hospital.

The focus group discussions were conducted to further clarify the data generated by the questionnaires and the interviews (Calder, 1980; Szybillo & Berger, 1979; Wells, 1974). Eight groups of nurses were randomly selected from the total population of nurses for participation in the focus groups, with seven or eight nurses in each group (n = 62). Each group evaluated one of six areas for improvement in the hospital that had been identified in the interviews. Q-sort methodology was used by group members to individually rank order suggestions for change within the hospital (Kerlinger, 1973). Once each member had completed ordering their list of suggestions, they reported and discussed their rankings with the rest of the group. Following group discussion, members re-evaluated their rankings and submitted them for tabulation by the group facilitator who presented the top areas for change to the group. The group then discussed the top-rated suggestions and examined strategies for implementing these changes.

Assessment Results

The questionnaire administration generated a response rate of 76% (n = 408). The climate scale data represented the overall hospital communication climate as being unexceptional, neither highly positive nor negative. (The mean score for all climate items was 2.9 on a 1 to 5 scale, where 1 = highly positive and 5 = highly negative.) The climate subscale of administrative recognition was rated as being most negative (3.3), while staff congruence and facility conditions were in the neutral range (2.8). The job satisfaction scale data indicated a slightly above average overall level of job satisfaction among nurses, with a mean score of 30.1 out of a possible 48, and 26.6 being set by past research as the neutral point (Smith, Kendall, & Hulin, 1969). The satisfaction subscale of promotions was rated as the greatest dissatisfier (19.1 with a neutral point of 20), pay as the next greatest dissatisfier (21.3 with a neutral point of 22), and coworkers as the greatest satisfier (40.1 with a neutral point of 32). Work was rated as the next greatest satisfier (32.7 with a neutral point of 26), and supervision was rated as mildly satisfying (37.3 with 33 as the neutral point).

The interview research phase elaborated upon the data generated by the questionnaire, with interviewers using open-ended questions and probing for in-depth answers to questions about strengths and weaknesses of work-life at the hospital and urging respondents to suggest specific areas for improvement within the hospital. The 49 interviews generated 875 suggestions for improving the hospital. Through content analysis the 875 suggestions were grouped topically into 6 general areas for change: benefits, communication, education, environment, organizational structure, and supplies and equipment. Each of the 6 general topic areas was composed of between 8 and 13 specific recommendation headings. For example, within the communication topic area the 13 recommendation headings were: improve administrative communication, improve feedback and recognition, improve interdepartmental communication, improve communication in nursing service, personalize communication, communicate nursing roles and responsibilities, improve hospital communication channels, improve public relations communication, improve attitudes and negative tone of communications, improve nurse-doctor communication, improve decision-making communication, increase information to administration about nursing needs, and improve communication within departments. Within each recommendation heading, on each of the six topic areas, specific recommendations (from the 875 suggestions offered) were listed.

In the focus group discussions, results from the interviews and the questionnaires were examined, evaluated, and rated (as to their importance) by groups of nurses. The rankings for the recommendation headings on each of the six topic areas were tabulated, and the twenty highest rated recommendation headings overall were compiled. (These recommendations are specific to the hospital under investigation and are not intended to be generalized to other hospitals or other organizations.)

Translating Assessment into Organizational Development

The goal of assessment was to collect interpretive organizational data to be used in establishing organizational development intervention strategies for relieving the problem of excessive nurse turnover facing the hospital. Data gathered through the three research phases were used to identify specific concerns nurses had about the hospital, and an ongoing retention organizational development program was implemented to relieve these concerns, encourage nurses to stay on their jobs, and improve organizational performance. A retention committee composed of representatives was formed from different areas and levels within nursing service at the hospital. The goals of the retention committee were to examine the specific problem areas, concerns, and suggestions generated through the research, to seek additional information about the issues identified, and to provide recommendations to hospital decision makers to initiate informed interventions and increase nurse retention at the hospital. The retention committee was designed to perform an important communicative role within the organization by providing a two-way information link between nursing staff and hospital administration.

Some of the specific communicative activities of the retention committee members were to bring information to the committee to act upon, identify and report on additional concerns of nurses, circulate information from the committee to hospital employees, and report on personal information about nursing staff (such as births, graduations, marriages, etc.) to the committee to be published in the retention newsletter, "Dialogue." The newsletter was designed to provide nursing staff with information about the activities of the retention committee, including issues under consideration and innovations being implemented, as well as to provide a channel for nurses to express their concerns about the hospital to other staff members. Personal news about staff members is reported in the newsletter as a way to share interesting information among nurses, as well as to promote a sense of hospital identification among staff members.

The retention organizational development program was designed to identify recurring problems facing nursing staff that lead to job dissatisfaction and turnover. The data gathered were used to implement specific action plans to resolve recurring problems. The retention committee and the newsletter were introduced to initiate action upon the problems identified and provide feedback between nursing staff and hospital administration. The retention committee represented all hospital nurses as an information clearinghouse, helping to preserve organizational intelligence possessed by nurses and use that intelligence for directing organizational development. The retention program established formal communication channels for nurses to provide administration with information about specific organizational problems and how they can be solved. It empowers nurses to air their gripes and direct the development of new hospital policies and practices.

Evaluation of the Retention Organizational Development Program

The retention program was implemented in early 1982 and has been monitored and evaluated for its first three years of operation. The retention program became a permanent structural innovation in the hospital, and the full effect of the program on the organization may not be apparent for many years. Certainly measurable changes in employee attitudes due to such an intervention in a large complex organization will take time to emerge. Additionally, socioeconomic environmental constraints that influence hospitals, such as inflation, budget allocations, workload, administrative changes, etc., will undoubtedly influence nurse turnover at the hospital. Nonetheless, interesting changes in hospital policies, practices, and nurse retention patterns have been observed and measured since the implementation of the nurse retention organizational development program.

Archival measures of institutional records of the rate of nurse turnover have been "unobtrusively" monitored in the hospital before and after the introduction of the retention program (Webb, et al., 1966). These data indicate the retention program may indeed have had a positive influence on nurse retention at the hospital. During 1981 (the year before the retention program was implemented) the nurse turnover rate was 35%; during 1982 (the first year of the program) the turnover rate dropped 2% to 33%; during 1983 (the second year of the program) the turnover rate dropped 4% more to 29%; and during 1984 (the third year of the program) the turnover rate dropped 2% more to 27%. Nurse retention improved by 8% during the first three years the retention organizational development program has been in operation.

These retention figures must be evaluated cautiously. There may be unexplained variance that is influencing this reduction in nurse turnover at the hospital. To control for some of the environmental factors influencing turnover rates at the hospital during the four year period, 1981 through 1984, unobtrusive archival records of turnover rates were examined at four comparable large urban full-service hospitals in the same Midwestern city. These turnover rates were compared with the reductions in turnover observed in the hospital where the retention program had been implemented. None of the four comparable hospitals had experienced as high a reduction in turnover between 1981 and 1984 as the retention program hospital had. The highest three-year reduction in turnover among any of the four comparison hospitals was 2.6% as contrasted with the turnover reduction of 8% at the retention program hospital over the same time period. Overall, the four comparison hospitals averaged a reduction in nurse turnover of .8% contrasted with a 2% reduction at the retention program hospital between 1981 and 1982, as well as a reduction of 1.3% contrasted with 4% between 1982 and 1983, and a change in turnover of +1.3% as contrasted with -2% between 1983 and 1984. (See Table 1 for these comparison turnover reduction figures.) These data indicate that, controlling for similar environmental influences, the retention program hospital experienced higher reductions of turnover than the four comparable urban hospitals. This adds strength to the contention that the retention organizational development program did help the hospital where it was implemented reduce turnover and increase retention of nursing staff.

Table 1

Comparison of Changes in Turnover Between the Research Hospital and Four Comparable Hospitals

	1981-1982	1982-1983	1983-1984	Total Change
Research Hospital	-2%	-4%	-2%	-8%
Average of Four Comparable Hospitals	-.8%	-1.3%	+1.3%	-.8%

Nurses' responses to job satisfaction and communication climate scales before and after the implementation of the retention organizational development program revealed less than the actual retention rates in evaluating the impact of the retention program on the hospital. Two follow-up questionnaires about the communication climate and job satisfaction were conducted at the hospital six months and twelve months after the introduction of the retention program to identify any changes in nurses' ratings of climate and satisfaction. No significant differences in overall ratings of satisfaction and climate between the three questionnaires were detected, indicating that job-satisfaction and communication climate are relatively stable organizational characteristics that have not been strongly influenced by the retention program at this time, but may change in the future. There is not a strong correlation between job satisfaction and attitudes about the climate with the actual measured retention rates.

Unstructured interviews with selected members of the nursing staff and hospital administration (n = 27; 24 nurses and 3 administrators) were conducted after the third year the retention program had been in operation to determine these individuals' reactions to the retention organizational development program. The respondents strongly indicated that members of the hospital perceive the retention program as a productive innovation in the organization. Virtually all nurses surveyed responded that they felt better about the hospital and their jobs because of the opportunity provided them by the retention program to voice their concerns about the hospital and participate in the hospital's organizational decision-making process. Those hospital administrators who were interviewed reported that meaningful dialogue between nurses, as well as between nurses and administrators, had increased as a result of the communication channels afforded them in the retention program. In addition it was reported that the retention program had been instrumental in initiating several problem-solving innovations within the hospital including: new in-service education programs (including cross-disciplinary and interdepartmental educational programs), a clinical nursing career ladder, improvement of child-care facilities available to nurses, and introduction of exit interview procedures for nurses. The retention program has also served to redefine the recruitment activities of members of the nursing administration to incorporate several retention, counseling, and staff development responsibilities. Moreover, the retention organizational development program has served to legitimize the relevant information nurses possess about hospital functioning and to develop mechanisms for utilizing this information to help improve the organization.

An important aspect of this study is that there was no set formula for solving the problem of nurse turnover and there was no simple reason for turnover that can be applied to the turnover problems experienced in other organizations. Rather than introducing predetermined intervention programs and strategies into the hospital, the retention program was designed to respond to the specific conditions of the organization under investigation by seeking organization-specific information from hospital nurses and using these data to guide innovations. This implies that there is no one set solution for solving excessive nurse turnover. Each hospital must be studied independently and organizational development strategies established for its specific organizational needs.

This study also illustrates the importance of developing organizational reflexivity in hospitals and other organizations (Kreps, 1985; 1986). The ability of hospital administrations to see their organization the way their employees do can help these leaders recognize and resolve pressing organizational problems. Additionally, a program that legitimizes employees' interpretations of organizational reality and uses the information they provide can increase individual commitment and involvement with the organization and jobs. By helping to solve organizational problems, these organization members can develop pride in their participation in organizational development. In hospitals, nurses can be given more opportunities to participate in organizational decision making, and the information they provide can help solve the specific problems they face daily on their jobs. In this study, organizational reflexivity was enhanced to help reduce nurse turnover, increase nurse retention, and develop organizational development strategies and programs to help improve the health care organization.

References

Albrecht, T. L. & Ropp, V. A. 1982. The study of network structuring in organizations through the use of method triangulation. *Western Journal of Speech Communication*, 46, 162-78.

Calder, B. 1980. Focus group interviews and qualitative research in organizations. In E. Lawler, D. Nodler, & C. Cammann (eds.), *Organizational assessment: Perspectives on the measurement of organizational behavior and the quality of work life*, 399-417. New York: John Wiley and Sons.

Filoromo, T. & Ziff, D. 1980. *Nurse recruitment: Strategies for success*. Rockville, MD: Aspen Systems Corporation.

French, W. L., Bell, C. H., & Zawacki, R. A. 1978. *Organizational development: Theory, practice, and research*. Dallas: Business Publications.

Hunter, R. E. 1978. *The mental health center climate questionnaire*. Paper presented to the International Communication Association conference, Chicago.

Hunter, R. E. 1976. *The development and evaluation of an organizational climate questionnaire for mental health centers*. Unpublished doctoral dissertation, Ohio University, Athens.

Jick, T. 1979. Mixing qualitative and quantitative methods: Triangulation in action. *Administrative Science Quarterly*, 24, 602-11.

Kerlinger, F. N. 1973. *Foundations of behavioral research*, second edition. New York: Holt, Rinehart, and Winston Incorporated.

Knight, K. E. & McDaniel, R. R. 1979. *Organizations: An information systems perspective*. Belmont, CA: Wadsworth.

Kreps, G. L. 1986. *Organizational communication: Theory and Practice*. White Plains, NY: Longman Incorporated.

Kreps, G. L. 1985. Organizational communication and organizational effectiveness. *World Communication*, 14, 109-19.

Kreps, G. L. 1983. *Organizational communication and organizational culture: A Weickian perspective*. Paper presented to the Academy of Management conference, Dallas.

Kreps, G. L. & Thornton, B. C. 1984. *Health communication: Theory and Practice*. New York: Longman Incorporated.

Lippitt, G. 1973. *Visualizing change*. Fairfax, VA: NTL Learning Resources Corporation.

Mobley, W. 1982. Some unanswered questions about turnover and withdrawal research. *Academy of Management Review*, 7, 111-16.

Mobley, W. 1977. Intermediate linkages in the relationship between job satisfaction and employee turnover. *Journal of Applied Psychology*, 67, 237-40.

Rogers, E.M. & Agarwala-Rogers, R. 1978. *Communication in organizations*. New York: The Free Press.

Salem, P. & Williams, M. L. 1984. Uncertainty and satisfaction: The importance of information in hospital communication. *Journal of Applied Communication Research*, 12, 75-89.

Smith, P. C., Kendall, L. M., & Hulin, C. L. 1969. *The measurement of satisfaction in work and retirement: A strategy for the study of attitudes*. Chicago: Rand McNally & Company.

Szybillo, G. J. & Berger, R. 1979. What advertising agencies think of focus groups. *Journal of Advertising Research*, 19, 29-33.

Wandelt, M. A., Pierce, P. M., and Widdowson, R. R. 1981. Why nurses leave nursing and what can be done about it. *American Journal of Nursing*, 81, 72-77.

Webb, E. J., Campbell, D. T., Schwartz, R. D. & Sechrist, L. 1966. *Unobtrusive measures: Nonreactive research in the social sciences*. Chicago: Rand McNally & Company.

Weick, K. E. 1979. *The social psychology of organizing*, second edition. Reading, MA: Addison-Wesley.

Wells, W. D. 1974. Group interviewing. In R. Ferber (ed.), *Handbook of Marketing Research*, 2-133, 2-146. New York: McGraw-Hill.

Wolf, G. A. 1981. Nursing turnover: Some causes and solutions. *Nursing Outlook*, April issue, 233-36.

CHAPTER
6

Health Communication Messages and Media

One of the most important goals of modern health care is to disseminate relevant and persuasive health information to health care providers and consumers to reduce health risks and promote public health. Providers need timely and accurate health information to keep up-to-date with advances in diagnosis and treatment of health problems in order to recognize health threats and to provide the best health care services to their clients. Consumers need relevant health information about strategies they can use to resist imminent health threats and respond to current health problems. Providing relevant health information to those people who most need such information is a major communication challenge to health care professionals.

While communication is a primary tool for accomplishing public health promotion, such communication must be strategically designed to reach and influence specific targeted audiences for health promotion. Messages have to be tailored to specific audiences to reflect audience needs, interests, and communication characteristics. The specific language used in health promotion messages and the organization of health promotion presentations must be designed to capture audience members' attention, evoke their understanding of the health issues described, and persuade them to adopt risk-preventing and health-promoting behaviors. Moreover, health promotion dissemination media must be selected carefully to both reach and influence specific target audiences. For example, attempting to influence the health behaviors of heroin addicts by advertising in the *Wall Street Journal* will obviously fail to adequately reach and influence this population because this newspaper is probably not their prime medium of choice.

There are many different channels available for health promotion communication. Health care providers can educate their clients about health risks and health promoting behaviors in personal interviews. In fact, interpersonal communication channels are often very influential sources of health information. Printed pamphlets, booklets, posters, and flyers are popular, and relatively inexpensive, health promotion media. Public presentations for interested groups can be an effective information dissemination medium. Telephone hot-lines (toll-free numbers) have also been used successfully to personally and anonymously provide relevant health information and social support to people in need of help (Kreps & Thornton, 1992).

Public mass media (such as radio, television, films, magazines, and newspapers) are probably the most powerful communication channels for reaching large audiences. News media have become increasingly popular channels for disseminating health information, yet are often not as well attended to as entertainment media. Entertainment media are an especially attractive communication channel for most people, and therefore can be very influential in helping to form public health beliefs and expectations. Unfortunately, current evidence suggests that entertainment media are not often used effectively to promote health and, in fact, often provide inaccurate health information to the public. New electronic computerized media (such as on-line information services, CD-ROM indexes, interactive computer programs, and e-mail hotlines) have become increasingly popular new channels for health information dissemination. This section of the book provides an examination of the use of both entertainment media and computer systems to disseminate health information to relevant publics.

The first reading in this chapter "Curing Television's Ills: The Portrayal of Health Care," is an article originally published in the *Journal of Communication* by Joe Turow and Lisa Coe. They report a content analytic study of the ways that popular television shows portray health care. As you review this article, think about the implications of television coverage of health care for public attitudes about personal health and health care treatment. The data presented about the portrayal of illnesses, consumers, and providers of health care is fascinating. For example, note the fact that there were very few elderly consumers of health care represented in the sampled television shows, about 5%, even though the aged are actually one of the largest populations of health care consumers in modern society. How are physicians, nurses, and other allied health care providers represented? What influence, if any, do you think the kinds of television coverage reported in this study has on public attitudes and health behaviors?

The second reading in this chapter "Disseminating Cancer Treatment Information to Physicians," was written by Gary Kreps and is a case study of the development, organization, and formative evaluation of a computer-based cancer treatment information dissemination system, the Physician Data Query (PDQ) system. This system is a good example of the use of new communication technologies such as interactive media to promote public health. This computer information system is designed to help physicians who care for cancer patients keep up-to-date with the latest scientific information concerning cancer treatment, optimally encouraging these physicians to learn about and adopt the most effective cancer treatment strategies available. Is a computer format a good way to disseminate this information? Can you think of some advantages and limitations to using a computer-based communication channel to disseminate cancer treatment information? Who, in addition to cancer treatment physicians, do you think might benefit from the information contained on the PDQ system?

Kreps, G. L. & Thornton, B. C. (1992). *Health Communication: Theory and Practice* 2nd edition. Prospect Heights, IL: Waveland Press.

13

Curing Television's Ills
The Portrayal of Health Care
By *Joseph Turow* and *Lisa Coe*

Much writing about television's depictions of health care takes as its starting point a concern that the medium be used to inculcate good health habits among children and adults (Hamburg & Pierce, 1982; Solomon, 1982). There is, however, another approach to TV's contribution to health care, one that demands a different kind of program analysis. It is that beneath any concerns for health education lie broader notions about the medical institution's power to define, prevent, and treat illness in society (see Gandy, 1981).

This latter view argues that U.S. network television's major contribution to public perceptions of health lies in outlining the accepted and the contested options for professional health care and in repeating dramatically, through news and entertainment, lessons about for whom society should care, why, when, and how. It is to this shared national agenda that politicians most strongly feel a need to respond publicly when formulating health care policy. When certain issues do not make TV's ledger, politicians feel less compulsion to reach a national consensus about the problems and more of an incentive either to ignore them or to flow with solutions demanded by special interests.

While a number of significant contributions have been made toward advancing this perspective, no systematic issue-guided analysis of TV programming exists that can be used as a platform for inquiring more deeply into the medium's implications for the health care system's structure and power. Our study represents one step in this direction. Specifically, we inquire into the extent to which profound changes that have transformed the U.S. medical system during the past decade have found contemporary expression in the treatment of illness on network TV. The analysis of a large block of network television news, entertainment, and commercials reveals a huge gap between actual changes in the structure of medical care and TV's portrayal of that

Reprinted with permission from the *Journal of Communication*, 1985, 35(4), 36-51. Dr. Turow is a professor in the Annenberg School for Communication at the University of Pennsylvania. Ms. Coe is an Account Executive at Fleishman Communications, Palatine, Illinois.

structure. The findings raise important questions about the consequences of this disjuncture for public policy. In addition, they raise the more general and hardly examined issue of the mass media's coverage of institutional change.

Public and private policy making on medical issues during the past decade and a half have been propelled by two major considerations: the increasing relative importance of chronic as opposed to acute illnesses, and the rising costs of U.S. medical care in relation to other segments of the economy. The first consideration, chronic or long-term illness, has been characterized by the Robert Wood Johnson Foundation as a "mounting problem," one of "the longer-term trends that will have a major influence on U.S. society's health care arrangements" (Annual Report, 1983, pp. 11-12, 16-17). A growing aged segment of the population, free from acute (short-term) problems (thanks, in part, to medical science), has survived to meet a panoply of chronic difficulties — cancer, heart disease, diabetes, senile dementia, and more. Too, the success of intensive care procedures in saving young and old people who would have died a few years earlier has resulted in a broad range of difficulties for those who have survived, their relatives, and their friends. To medical ethicists and a growing number of self-help organizations, the increased presence of chronically ill people underscores the importance of aiding all involved in taking into account the social and psychological, not only biomedical, aspects of an illness: from its discovery through critical care management, through the integration of the chronically ill person into a long-term institutional setting or (not uncommonly) into mainstream society.

The second area of major concern — the rising costs of medical care — is to a considerable extent related to the public and private expense of treating an aging population with chronic problems. But costs have outpaced inflation in all parts of the medical system. By the mid-1980s, health care was consuming 10 percent of the U.S. gross national product (Council on Long Range Planning and Development, 1984). Many government and business leaders considered the situation intolerable.

The root causes for the spiraling cost increases are a matter of acrid dispute (for a historical perspective, see Starr, 1983). Regardless, concern over rising health care costs has sparked two major approaches by government and big business that are changing the structure of U.S. medicine. The first approach limits federal Medicare payments to hospitals according to predetermined disease categories called diagnostic related groups (DRGs). For example, a hospital that admits a 68-year-old man with a specific heart problem would receive a certain amount to pay for that patient, whether it actually needs more or less. The Medicare program is limited to people 65 years and older, but a number of state governments, spurred on by big business and the insurance industry, have been trying to apply this cost-limiting idea to patients of all ages. While the DRG regulations and related rules are still evolving and their full implications are impossible to determine, it is clear that they inject new incentives into the physician-hospital relationship. Whereas until just a few years ago hospital administrators working in an era of broad insurance coverage encouraged physicians to use hospital technology liberally, the new DRG regulations have created an economy of scarcity that demands frugality on the hospital's part and creates an important tension between the hospital administration and attending physicians on the desired approach to patient evaluation and treatment. Administrators now encourage a kind of competition among doctors in their use of hospital resources, with the implication that physicians who hinder the hospital from profiting from patient care will not long retain admitting privileges (Golin, 1984; Sullivan, 1984).

The second major approach to cost containment, one used by both the public and private sector, encourages the growth of medical delivery systems with lower per patient costs than those of private physicians and general hospitals — for example, health maintenance organizations, independent practice associations, preferred provider organizations, outpatient surgical facilities, hospital-owned hotels for relatively low-cost patient recovery, and "doc in the box" quick medical care facilities. Each arrangement brings its own incentives and disincentives for certain approaches to patient care. The competitive environment has also led established hospitals in many areas to compete fiercely for patients (for example, middle-class pregnant women) whose ability to pay has not been shaped by declining federal and state payment schedules. The poor and unemployed are clearly not part of those target groups, and in a number of localities — Detroit and Tampa are two examples — the scarcity of resources for them has reached crisis proportions (Finley, 1984; Lefton, 1984).

The foregoing sketch implies that much of the public and private response to health care costs can be understood in terms of the twin concepts of scarcity and competition. Also implied is that health care decisions are interrelated at the societal level — that they have sociopolitical as well as individual implications. In an era in which the development of expensive technology is allowing people with chronic illnesses to live longer and (sometimes) better than ever before, defining medical care as a scarce resource raises moral and logistical, as well as economic, questions (Aaron & Swartz, 1984; Weil, 1984). The same is true about the new competitive environment that is changing the structure of care for acute and chronic problems. In the United States a variety of major forces representing big business, labor, the aged, organized medicine, and the hospital, insurance, pharmaceutical, and medical technology industries are grappling furiously at the federal and state levels over the emerging system and its outcome (Rust, 1984; Sandrick, 1984).

But to what extent does network television incorporate these debates over the changing dimensions of illness and the changing structures of health care into programming? To what extent are these new circumstances — the increased prominence of chronic illness, the approach to health care as a scarce resource, and the injection of private competition into the scene — shown to have consequences for the way sick people are handled in a variety of medical and nonmedical settings? What are the implications of these TV presentations for public and professional response to the dynamics and politics of change in the medical institution? The purpose of this study was to answer these questions.

Our way into the problem was to explore how "ill" people — individuals or collectivities depicted or talked about — are "treated" on television. We defined "treatment" broadly to mean any attempt by an individual or an organization to address an ill person's physical or emotional state, through medical or nonmedical means. Drawing on the widely cited definition by Parsons (1951), we defined "illness" on TV as the impairment of a person's bodily functions so as to adversely affect the performance of "normal" social roles. Chronic illness is bodily impairment that adversely affects normal roles for an unforeseeable length of time. Acute illness, by contrast, is depicted as having an end in sight, whether it is a cure or death resulting from the illness. Since TV portrayals can depict the progress and outcome of the same illness in a variety of ways, we designated an illness as acute or chronic only after noting the way it was handled in the context of an "illness episode."

An "illness episode" was our major unit of analysis. We defined it as the portrayal of any activity by an individual or organization toward an ill person (or collectivity) or of any activity by an ill person (or collectivity) toward an individual or organization. Also included in the notion of an illness episode were portrayals of two or more individuals discussing the way to cope with the illness of others.

The length of an illness episode was limited by definition to not more than the length of a scene or news story; a different scene meant a different illness episode. Because an illness episode by definition involved one dyad, entertainment scenes or news stories that noted the interaction of a number of ill and healthy people might yield several illness episodes. In addition, because an ill person might interact with a number of individuals or organizations during the course of a program, the person's illness episodes could accumulate into a string we called an "illness series." We expected that the more episodes that comprised an illness series, the more varied would be the attention devoted by TV to that specific person and problem.

We examined the treatment of illness on ABC, NBC, and CBS during the first two weeks of November of 1983. Focusing on one network a day in rotation, we videorecorded the morning news program, two hours of soap operas (on weekdays), the evening news, and prime time, all including commercials. Then, after testing the reliability of an extensive coding scheme based on the concept of an illness episode (Scott's Pi = .87 with two coders), we systematically noted those aspects of the episodes that would illuminate the way TV deals with the changing dimensions of illness and the changing structure of health care.

The examination of 90.5 hours of network television over 14 days revealed 723 interactions in which ill people appeared. Commercials contained 34 percent of the illness episodes and afternoon serials 18 percent. Prime time fictional programming contained 33 percent, with evening serials (such as "Dynasty" and "St. Elsewhere") having 11 percent, evening series 14 percent, and movies 8 percent. Evening news broadcasts accounted for only 3 percent of the illness episodes, while news magazines (morning and evening) accounted for 12 percent. No matter what the programming, though, illness tended to take center stage when it appeared. Overall, 639 or 88 percent of the inter- actions in which ill people took part revolved in some way around their maladies. This figure was 98 percent in commercials, 96 percent in evening news and serials, 92 percent in news magazines, 82 percent in afternoon serials, 74 per- cent in prime time series, and 71 percent in movies.

The 723 illness episodes involved 380 "patients," whose numbers varied greatly in the different program types. Commercials had a total of 245 patients; the evening news, 15; news magazines, 46; afternoon serials, 35; evening serials, 21; evening series, 32; and movies, 6.[1] When they could be determined, the demographics of the ill population were found to parallel those typically found on network TV: male (58 percent of the 296 whose sex could be noted), non-ethnic white (89 percent of the 281 whose ethnicity could be noted), and white collar (60 percent of the 84 whose occupation could be noted). Even though people over the age of 65 confront the highest illness-related expenses and the most major illnesses in U.S. society (Council on Long Range Planning and Development, 1984), only 5 percent of the 214 patients whose age could be determined were over 65.

We used 29 categories to encompass the problems that afflicted people in our TV sample. Table 1 presents the distribution of these illnesses in three ways. The first, a listing of the illnesses afflicting the 380 patients, is a straightforward measure of attention to medical problems on TV. The second, which lists the distribution of illnesses according to the 723 illness episodes, is perhaps a better indication of the programs' emphases on particular illnesses; patients with certain illnesses were more likely to be depicted in a greater number of illness episodes than were patients with other illnesses. The third way of depicting the distri- bution of illnesses on TV presents their occurrence in the 132 patients who appeared outside the commercials — that is, where the most serious illnesses tended to show up.

The first column in Table 1 shows that the most frequent illness to hit TV's population was the common cold (affecting 27 percent of patients), followed by headache/fever, skeletal-muscular problems, gastrointestinal discomforts, and arthritis. Together, these five illnesses affected 219 (58 percent) of the 380 patients. Not surprisingly, 204 of those 219 patients (93 percent) showed up in commercials for pharmaceuticals.[2]

A look at the 723 illness episodes changes the emphasis somewhat. The second column of Table 1 shows that cold symptoms still ranked first, comprising 16 percent of all the illness interactions. But following cold symptoms were mental illness, drug abuse, headache/fever, and trauma. While mental illness and drug abuse together were problems for only 4 percent of the patients, considerable attention was paid to those patients. For example, a total of 51 out of 72 episodes involving mental illness revolved around the main character

Table 1

Illnesses on sampled television programming

	Individual patients (n = 380) %	Illness episodes (n = 723) %	Individual patients, excl. commercials (n = 135) %
Cold symptoms	27	16	—
Headache/fever	16	9	—
Skeletal/muscular	5	6	8
Gastrointestinal	5	2	—
Arthritis	5	3	0.8
Hemorrhoids	4	2	—
Severe trauma (accidents, gunshot wounds)	4	7	11
Cuts, bruises	4	5	7
Mental illness	3	10	8
Heart problems	3	6	7
Leprosy	2	3	7
Alcoholism	2	3	1.5
Birth defects	2	1	5
Drug abuse	1	9	3
Eyesight problems	1	0.7	2
Transplant needed	1	2	4
Neurological problems	1	4	3
Cancer	1	1	3
Autoimmune problems	1	0.8	3
Poisoned	1	0.8	3
Lung problems	0.8	0.4	0.8
Appendicitis	0.8	0.4	2
Mental retardation	0.8	0.4	2
Anorexia nervosa	0.5	0.4	1.5
Diabetes	0.5	0.3	—
Malaria	0.5	1	1.5
Other	1	0.6	1.5
Mixed problems	1	0.8	1.5
Unspecified	4	5	11
Total	98.4[a]	100.6[a]	98.1[a]

[a]Rounding error

of *Ordinary People*, a two-and-a-half hour theatrical film aired by NBC.

Excluding commercials when looking at patients' illnesses highlights those illnesses depicted in television news and entertainment programs. The third column in Table 1 shows that, for the 135 patients not in advertisements, the most common illness was trauma. According to health experts, trauma is a major health problem in the United States, especially the kind of trauma that leads to chronic debilitation (Trunkey, 1983, p. 35; Vaughan, et al., 1979). In our sample, however, none of the 48 episodes that depicted trauma approached the problem as chronic. While 12 episodes took an unclear stance, the rest presented dramatic violence that led rapidly to cure or death. The next five most frequent illnesses in the noncommercial sample were skeletal/ muscular, mental illness, heart problems, cuts and bruises, and leprosy. (A chronic problem rare in the United States, leprosy was the focus of a segment of the news magazine "20/20" that depicted a leper colony in Hawaii.)

Heart problems and mental illness are also considered major problems by U.S. health experts. Although physicians generally regard both as having important chronic aspects (Ahmed & Coelho, 1979; Engel, 1981), of the 72 illness episodes that dealt with problems of heart or mind in news or entertainment, 40 (68 percent) dealt with the problem on an acute basis (for example, going into surgery or expressing the opinion that the emotional problem was temporary).

One example from the soap opera "The Young and the Restless" gives the flavor of TV's tendency to ignore the implications of long-term illness. A young adult woman in the program, Traci, overdosed on drugs and ended up in the hospital, where doctors found that she had severely damaged her heart. Eventually, they told her that she would have to take heart medicine for the rest of her life. After her release, however, that plot line was dropped and while the character was heard of again, her heart ailment was not.

Over the course of our two sampled weeks of "The Young and the Restless," Traci's problem was covered in 30 illness episodes, 23 of which treated her overdose as an acute difficulty (suggesting that she would be fully cured quickly) and only 7 as chronic. While Traci's story reflects the acute "tilt" of network TV's handling of illness, her illness series was quite unusual in that it was relatively long and portrayed the reactions of various people to her problem at various times. Many of her illness episodes involved agonized relatives discussing her problem among themselves or with doctors.

By contrast, most illness series in our sample did not have the potential for anything approaching the comparatively textured depiction of Traci's illness. This is because 85 percent of the 380 illness series involved only 1 illness episode, 95 percent involved 5 or fewer episodes, and only 3 series in the entire sample (including Traci's) exceeded 21 episodes. As Table 2 indicates, the three long illness series appeared in two afternoon serials (a drug abuse subplot on "As the World Turns" plus Traci's subplot on "The Young and the Restless") and one movie, *Ordinary People*, which focused on the difficulties of an

Table 2

Program types by length of illness series

	Short series (n = 360) %	Medium series (n = 17) %	Long series (n = 3) %
Evening news	4	—	—
News magazines	12	18	—
Prime time series	7	29	—
Afternoon serials	3	18	67
Evening serials	4	29	—
Movies	1	—	33
Commercials	69	6	—
Total	100	100	100

Note: A short series denotes 1-5 illness episodes; a medium series denotes 6-20 illness episodes; and a long series denotes 21 or more illness episodes. Within each row, all frequencies are significantly different by the chi-square test, with $p \leq .001$.

emotionally ill youngster. Table 3 indicates that afternoon serials and movies were also the program formats most likely to depict patients with "textured" medical problems — that is, problems shown to have both chronic and acute (or possibly uncertain) aspects to them. By contrast, commercials and news programs tended to zero in on patients more fleetingly than other program formats and were more likely to depict patients' problems as straightforward. In this sense, of course, the treatment of illness merely exaggerates a general characteristic of TV's program formats. Overall, only 21 (5 percent) of all patients had "textured" medical problems.

Of the 359 patients whose illnesses were depicted in an untextured manner, the short-term and the clear-cut carried the day, as Table 3 shows. Commercials, the program form with the largest number of patients, also had the largest number of patients with acute illnesses (to be alleviated by the advertised product), followed by news magazines, evening series, and afternoon serials. In both news magazines and the evening news, where items on birth defects, AIDS, leprosy, cerebral palsy, and cancer found air time, the percentages of "chronic only" stories were relatively high. Interestingly, none of the patients in afternoon serials or movies had their illnesses depicted as only chronic; the chronically sick people on soap operas typically had "textured" illness series.

Whether the problems they dealt with were portrayed as chronic or acute, all types of TV programming tended to emphasize biomedical (that is, pharmacological or technological) over interpersonal and psychological attempts to deal with illness. Of the 723 illness episodes, 66 percent involved the suggestion or performance of specific biomedical actions and only 10 percent

Figure 3 Illness Characteristics by Program Types (in Episodes)

	Evening news	News magazines	Prime-time series	Afternoon serials	Evening serials	Movies	Commercials	Total
"Medical texture" of illnesses	(n = 15) %	(n = 46) %	(n = 31) %	(n = 15) %	(n = 21) %	(n = 6) %	(n = 245) %	(n = 380) %
Textured	7	7	16	33	10	34	—	5
Untextured	93-	93	84	66	90	66	100	95
Total	100	100	100	99ᵃ	100	100	100	100
Nature of untextured illnesses	(n = 14) %	(n = 43) %	(n = 27) %	(n = 10) %	(n = 19) %	(n = 4) %	(n = 242) %	(n = 359) %
Acute only	50	42	49	50	68	50	83	72
Chronic only	36	44	29	—	33	—	10	16
Uncertain only	14	14	22	50	—	50	7	11
Total	100	100	100	100	101ᵃ	100	100	99ᵃ
Coping vs. biomedical in illness episodes	(n = 22) %	(n = 83) %	(n = 102) %	(n = 129) %	(n = 78) %	(n = 61) %	(n = 248) %	(n = 723) %
Coping	—	8	8	49	21	11	3	10
Biomedical	99	80	62	16	74	76	94	66
Other	1	12	30	35	5	13	3	24
Total	100	100	100	100	100	100	100	100
Location of illness episode (when known)	(n = 8) %	(n = 51) %	(n = 95) %	(n = 115) %	(n = 72) %	(n = 57) %	(n = 51) %	(n = 449) %
Hospital	88	47	36	67	74	5	10	43
Doctor's office	—	4	1	2	3	19	—	4
Other medical location	—	—	—	—	—	—	8	1
Dwelling	12	14	6	5	4	40	39	14
Other nonmedical location	—	35	57	26	19	35	43	38
Total	100	100	100	100	100	99ᵃ	100	100

Note: Within each row, all frequencies are significantly different by the chi-square test, with $p \leq .001$.   ᵃ Rounding error.

involved psychosocial coping (12 percent of episodes did not relate to the patient's illness at all and another 12 percent revolved around the illness in a general manner — describing it or making small talk in the hospital room). Only 2 of the 248 commercials referred to psychosocial coping. Of the 396 noncommercial illness episodes that revolved around illness, only 18 percent depicted psychological aspects of coping with the problem on the part of the patient, family, friends, or health professionals. Table 3 shows that afternoon serials had by far the highest percentage of coping episodes, with evening serials a distant second.

Psychosocial concerns about coping made up only 16 percent of the 205 discussions that relatives, strangers, and friends had with patients and only 5 percent of the 177 interactions between health professionals and patients. Other kinds of attempts at this aspect of coping were also infrequently portrayed. Only 43 of the 723 interactions revolving around ill people involved two individuals other than the patient discussing ways to handle the psychosocial consequences of illness. As for the 246 episodes that showed patients trying to cope with illness alone, 203 appeared on commercials, and they all ended with decisions to take drugs. Of the remaining 43 "patient alone" episodes, only 6 saw patients trying to cope psychologically with their own illness. One of these exceptions, on "St. Elsewhere," showed a heart patient listening to classical music to keep her mind off her upcoming transplant. Another, a news report on "Good Morning America," told of a cerebral palsy victim's decision to starve herself to death.

People with chronic problems were significantly more likely than people with acute illnesses to be involved in coping episodes (22 percent vs. 10 percent). However, an examination of the references to coping revealed that, for both chronic and acute illnesses, "coping" often (59 percent of 152 references) meant words of comfort or other efforts at short-term help rather than plans for long-term handling of the problem, plans that could be important in chronic diseases. Further, only 4 percent or 17 of the 475 noncommercial illness episodes depicted one or more patients returning to society. And, in line with TV's emphasis on clear-cut solutions, 12 of these 17 episodes depicted the problems as acute and only 4 as chronic.

In contrast to the rarity and superficiality of a psychosocial approach to illness, especially chronic illness, drugs and machines were ubiquitous as vehicles of healing. Pharmacological treatments were most common, comprising 54 percent of the 478 specific biomedical interventions. Following pharmacology in frequency were mechanical (such as traction — 15 percent), surgical (9 percent), diagnostic (4 percent), psychiatric (4 percent), nutritional (3 percent), and other (2 percent) approaches. Both pharmacological and technological approaches were scattered broadly through the news and entertainment programs, although there was an emphasis on the technological (especially the surgical) that was statistically significant. In commercials, however, solutions were almost exclusively related to drugs (91 percent).

Table 3 shows that of the 51 commercials whose locations could be ascertained, 39 percent took place in the person's home, 51 percent in some other nonmedical location, and 10 percent within a hospital. Commercials had an uncertain or uncodable location in 197 (79 percent) of 248 occurrences. Frequent demonstrations of self-medication can be inferred from these figures. By contrast, in news and entertainment collectively, of the 398 episodes that could be located (84 percent of the total), 52 percent took place in some part of a hospital. The prominence of the hospital did not differ substantially whether the illness was depicted as acute or chronic, but it did differ across program types. As Table 3 shows, hospital treatment of illness was especially prominent in the evening news, afternoon serials, and evening serials. It was least prominent in the evening series and the movies.

The point to underscore here is that in all programs the hospital showed overwhelming dominance as a location for the *professional* treatment of illness. As Table 3 indicates, only four percent of the illness episodes took place in any professional medical location other than a hospital. All but four of these locations were a doctor's office, and two of those involved a psychiatrist's room in the film *Ordinary People*. This means that, aside from four local ads for a drug dependency center, commercials, news, and fictive entertainment ignored the various kinds of long-term and intermediate care facilities, the numerous forms of nonhospital outpatient surgical or ambulatory facilities, the various types of nonspecialist private practice locations, and the numerous kinds of health maintenance organizations that exist throughout the country. Also ignored were many kinds of medical personnel aside from hospital-based doctors and nurses. Excluding commercials (where only 4 medical professionals appeared and occupations in general were mostly unknown), medical professionals appeared in 214 (56 percent) of the 379 interactions in which occupations were known. Of those 214, 70 percent were physicians, 13 percent were nurses, and 16 percent made up all other categories of health care personnel.

The so-called allied health professions were sparsely and indistinctly represented. Only 11 episodes in entertainment programming depicted practicing medical professionals other than doctors and nurses. Three of these showed ambulance drivers/paramedics, two a physical therapist, one a nutritionist, one an X-ray technician, and the rest persons who fit into only the vague occupational category of "medical personnel." The same vagueness characterized the 12 news spots and 14 commercials in which "other medical personnel" appeared. Optometrists in Sears' optical department ads and, in the news, an occupational therapist, a hospital spokesperson, and an organ transplant coordinator were the only specific jobs that could be noted. Missing entirely from television were nurse practitioners and physician assistants, two controversial and relatively new occupational categories that are having an impact on the structure of primary medical care in the United States (Cousins, 1979).

Medical care itself was portrayed as overwhelmingly appropriate, nonpolitical, and as an unlimited resource. In the 174 circumstances where medical professionals gave specific biomedical orders or carried out biomedical tasks, they were clearly correct in 78 percent of the cases and incorrect in only 3 percent (2 percent of the cases showed a mixed result and in 14 percent the result was indeterminate). Arguments about the giving of specific biomedical care occurred in only 7 of the 723 illness episodes and dealt with three cases. Two of these were issues in the news: the decision by physicians and parents not to operate to keep a congenitally malformed infant (a "Baby Doe") alive, and the refusal of staff physicians in another city to allow a cerebral palsy patient to starve herself to death in their hospital. The third was the start of a subplot in the prime time medical serial "St. Elsewhere" that dealt with the desire of a surgeon to perform a heart transplant and the refusal of the city's hospital administrator to allow it for cost reasons. This last illness series was the only one in our sample that dealt with scarce resources. Although broached, the subject was treated quite gingerly and narrowly. At issue was not whether another transplant could be done at all, but whether it could be done at that hospital when other hospitals in the city had been designated previously as transplant centers.

Note, too, that in the few instances in which politics was involved in our TV sample of medical care, it related exclusively to the moral and legal obligations that physicians confront when they treat patients lingering on the edge of life. By contrast, contemporary medical periodicals are rife with examples of how politics in the medical system affects patient care at all stages of illness. The cumulative picture one gets in the medical trade literature — and in recent sociological writings on medicine — is that current political and economic battles are having complex and widespread impacts on the contours of the health of the U.S. population and on the very definitions of illness and health. Yet this key realization found no echo in our TV sample. Instead, news, entertainment, and advertising enacted the quite opposite notion that medical care is an apolitical, unlimited resource, available to all through either quick-acting drugs or economically stable acute care hospitals.

The dominant pattern of illness portrayal in our sample did not confront today's most enduring medical problems. Overall, network television presented illness as acute and amenable to biomedical treatment. Illness episodes emphasized the short-term and the straightforward. Even when coping was discussed, the patient's long-range plans or reintegration into society was rarely considered.

There were, however, noteworthy differences between program formats on this matter. Afternoon serials and news programs tended to deal with chronic problems and coping much more than commercials and evening serials or series. Similarly, afternoon serials depicted psychosocial aspects of coping (short-term though they were) a good deal more often than the other formats. And, amid all the programming, the theatrical film *Ordinary People* stood out as a startling exception to the typical flow.

It seems likely that different dramatic conventions and production constraints guided the different tendencies of the TV formats toward or away from chronic problems. News programs focus on illnesses that reflect social or personal conflict. Chronic problems become news targets when they tie into biomedical or legal issues and can be encapsulated into short-term, life-or-death drama (see Winsten, pp. 20-27). The serial format lends itself to the portrayal of illness as chronic because of its continuing story line. In afternoon soap operas the likelihood of chronicity is increased because hospital sets are useful locations for necessarily low-budget productions (Cassata, 1979). Prime time series, on the other hand, have large budgets, more outdoor locales, and the need to wrap up loose ends within a sixty-minute plot. That discourages portrayals of chronic illness. So does the commercial format, since persuasive appeals for nonprescription drugs are likely to imply quick cure.

Finally, movies allow the possibility of a chronic focus because they have more time than typical programs and because their "one-shot" nature means that truly serious problems can befall central characters.[3] In addition, movie producers feel that they must attract audiences by promoting their works as unusual. So, when the creators decide to focus on illness, they have an incentive to feature problems that are controversial and difficult to solve, whether in a "disease of the week" heroic tale or in an exposé of a taboo subject, such as a youngster's mental illness.

While differences between program formats showed up regarding the dimensions of illness, they were starkly absent when it came to sociopolitical considerations. This study found that all the program formats overwhelmingly failed to confront the government and corporate activities that have been changing the contemporary medical system and the public's relationship to it. One road to uncovering the reasons for this failure might lie in considering the relationship that television networks and production firms have had with mainstream elements of the medical system. We can suggest that the relationship has been symbiotic, benefitting all parties. Over time, it has led to formats and formulas that have entrenched certain perspectives about the role of U.S. medicine on TV news, entertainment, and commercials. While the medical world has been changing drastically since those perspectives were set, neither side in the relationship to this point has seen fit to encourage change in the basic approaches to TV's depictions. For the networks and production firms, the standard approach works: it draws requisite audiences efficiently. For the medical establishment, government officials, business executives, and other contending interest groups, the standard approach ensures their continued acceptance by the broad audiences of the nation's most shared medium.

It may well be, then, that a key consequence of television's contemporary treatment of illness for the medical institution has been to encourage the belief of vested interests that they can negotiate key structural changes in the medical institution outside of the glare of network television. This study represents an inquiry into network television's message system during only one period, albeit a formative one, in the development of the contemporary medical structure. Network television's depictions are not static, and one might well expect that as time goes on indications of the changes will appear in fiction and nonfiction programming. However, the findings here suggest that depiction of the most critical changes will be reflected on network TV only after they have become entrenched politically. For the general public, particularly those who receive the bulk of their knowledge about medical trends from television, the consequence of this eventuality would seem to be the perpetuation in medicine of what Touraine (1971) calls "dependent participation:" involvement in and dependence upon institutional processes without knowing how and when powerful contending special interests have set the basic rules.

These possibilities hold many important implications for the role U.S. network television plays in a profoundly important aspect of institutional change. For the benefit of both theory and practice, they deserve further study.

Notes

[1] The number of patients appearing in commercials was large compared to the numbers on other types because all but three of the commercial illness episodes dealt with different people. By contrast, a few entertainment and news programs depicted the same patients across a large number of illness episodes. It might also be underscored that this study was conducted during November, a typical time for the common cold. Perhaps products to alleviate "cold symptoms" and "headache/fever" are particularly evident on TV during this time.

[2] Of the 380 patients, 199 (52 percent) stood out as individuals, while 181 (48 percent) were collectivities, that is, specific groups of patients (e.g., lepers in a colony in Hawaii) or general abstractions (e.g., people with head colds). The large number of collectivities might be taken to mean that programs consistently dealt with illness on broad intellectual, perhaps even sociopolitical, terms. This was not the case, however, since 159 (88 percent) of the collectivities appeared in commercials as mere surrogates for consumers of the persuasive message.

[3] This generalization does not apply to TV movies that are series pilots, since producers' intentions there are to spin the main characters off into their own weekly vehicles.

References

Aaron, Henry J. and William Schwartz. 1984. *The Painful Prescription: Rationing Hospital Care.* Washington, DC: Brookings Institution.

Ahmed, Paul and George Coelho (eds.). 1979. *Toward a New Definition of Health.* New York and London: Plenum.

Caplan, Arthur, H. Tristam Engelhardt, Jr., and James McCartney (eds.). 1981. *Concepts of Health and Disease.* Reading, MA: Addison-Wesley.

Cassata, Mary B., Thomas Skill, and Samuel Osei Boadu. 1979. "In Sickness and in Health." *Journal of Communication* 29(4), Autumn, pp. 73-80.

Cook, Fay Lomax et al. 1983. "Media and Agenda Setting: Effect on the Public, Interest Group Leaders, and Policy Makers." *Public Opinion Quarterly* 47(16), Spring, pp. 16-25.

Council on Long Range Planning and Development. 1984. *The Environment of Medicine*. Chicago: American Medical Association.

Cousins, Norman. 1979. *Anatomy of an Illness as Perceived by the Patient*. New York: Bantam.

"Detroit Community Hospital Faces May 31 Rescue Deadline." *American Medical News* 27(19), May 18, 1984, p. 39.

Engel, George. 1981. "The Need for a New Medical Model: A Challenge to Biomedicine." In Arthur Caplan, H. Tristam Engelhardt, Jr., and James McCartney (eds.), *Concepts of Health and Disease*. Reading, MA: Addison-Wesley.

Finley, Thomas. "Concerted Effort Needed to Control Health Costs." *American Medical News* 27(11), March 16, 1984, pp. 18-19.

"Former HEW Secretary Says Chrysler's Health Care Costs Too High." *American Medical News* 27(10), March 9, 1984, p. 28.

Gandy, Oscar. 1981. *Beyond Agenda Setting*. Norwood, NJ: Ablex.

Gerbner, George. 1974. "Teacher Image in Mass Culture: Symbolic Functions of the 'Hidden Curriculum'." In David Olson (ed.), *Media and Symbols*. Chicago: National Society for the Study of Education/University of Chicago Press.

Gerbner, George, Michael Morgan, and Nancy Signorielli. 1982. "Programming Health Portrayals." In David Pearl, Lorraine Bouthilet, and Joyce Lazar (eds.), *Television and Behavior*, 1982, Volume 2. Rockville, MD: National Institute of Mental Health.

Golin, Carol. "Trouble Ahead for MDs, Hospitals." *American Medical News* 27(18), May 11, 1984, pp. 3, 41-42.

Hamburg, Beatrix and Chester Pierce. 1982. "Television and Health: Introductory Comments." In David Pearl, Lorraine Bouthilet, and Joyce Lazar (eds.), *Television and Behavior*, 1982, Volume 2. Rockville, MD: National Institute of Mental Health.

Krause, Elliot. 1977. *Power and Illness*. New York: Elsevier.

Lefton, Doug. "Public Hospital Limits Care to Tampa's Poor." *American Medical News* 27(15), April 20, 1984, pp. 1, 23-24.

Lefton, Doug. "FTC Probe in Arizona: Did Hospitals Pressure Honeywell?" *American Medical News* 27(22), June 8, 1984, pp. 1, 24.

Lefton, Doug. "In Competition with Private Hospitals, Public Hospitals Go After Private Patients." *American Medical News* 27(26), July 13, 1984, p. 10.

McIlrath, Sharon. "MDs Targeted by Budget Trimming Efforts." *American Medical News* 27(13), April 6, 1984, pp. 28-29.

McIlrath, Sharon. "DRGs Seen Boosting Outpatient Care, Competition." *American Medical News* 27(24), June 22, 1984, p. 14.

Parsons, Talcott. 1951. *The Social System*. New York: Free Press.

Pellegrino, Edmund. 1979. "The Sociocultural Impact of Twentieth Century Therapeutics." In Morris Vogel and Charles R. Rosenberg (eds.), *The Therapeutic Revolution*. Philadelphia: University of Pennsylvania Press.

Robert Wood Johnson Foundation. 1983. *Annual Report*. Princeton, NJ: Robert Wood Johnson Foundation.

Rust, Mark. "Ethicists Devoting Increased Attention to Financial Issues." *American Medical News* 27(26), July 13, 1984, pp. 3, 43.

Rust, Mark. "New Medical Economics Are Emerging." *American Medical News* 27(26), July 13, 1984, pp. 41-42.

Sandrick, Karen. "Supportive Care Guidelines Stir Debate." *American Medical News* 27(20), May 25, 1984, pp. 3, 23-25.

Solomon, Douglas. "Health Campaigns on Television." In David Pearl, Lorraine Bouthilet, and Joyce Lazar (eds.), *Television and Behavior*, 1982, Volume 2. Rockville, MD: National Institute of Mental Health.

Starr, Paul. 1983. *The Social Transformation of American Medicine*. New York: Basic Books.

"State Seeks Reinstatement of Balance Billing Plan." *American Medical News* 27(15), April 20, 1984, pp. 1, 45.

Sullivan, Tony. "DRGs Spur New Player on Team." *American Medical News* 27(4), January 27, 1984, pp. 3, 21-22.

Swartz, Donald. "Dealing with Chronic Illness in Childhood." *Pediatrics in Review* 6(3), September 1984, pp. 67-73.

Touraine, Alain. 1971. *The Post-Industrial Society*. New York: Random House.

Trunkey, Donald. "Trauma." *Scientific American* 249(2), August 1983, pp. 28-35.

Vaughan, Victor, R. James McKay, and Richard E. Berman (eds.). 1979. *Nelson Textbook of Pediatrics* (11th ed.). Philadelphia: Saunders.

Weil, Max. "Boom in Critical Care Raises Economic, Ethical Dilemmas." *Emergency Medicine*, February 1984.

Winsten, Jay A. "Science and the Media: Telling the Truth." *Health Affairs*, in press. (Manuscript available from the author at the Harvard School of Public Health.)

Wohl, Sidney. 1984. *The Medical-Industrial Society*. New York: Harmony Books.

14

Disseminating Cancer Treatment Information to Physicians
The Case of the Physician Data Query (PDQ) System
By Gary L. Kreps

The PDQ Information System

The "PDQ" (Physician Data Query) information system is a relatively new on-line computerized database developed and administered by the National Cancer Institute (NCI) to disseminate state-of-the-art clinical cancer research and practice information from the cancer research community to the cancer treatment community (NCI, 1984). "The PDQ information system was developed to help physicians who see cancer patients keep abreast of the latest research data about successful techniques and settings for cancer care, and by doing so, improve the prognosis for the nation's cancer patients" (Sondik and Maibach, 1984, p. 368). PDQ uses a "user-friendly" (menu-driven) computer operating system designed to make information in the database accessible to both novice and experienced end-users (computer searchers) by eliminating the need for users to learn a specialized searching language.

In March of 1984, the NCI made the PDQ database available to the medical community at more than 2,000 medical libraries and health care institutions in the United States through the National Library of Medicine's (NLM) MEDLARS computer system (Culliton, 1985). Additionally, physicians can request an access code for PDQ from the NCI to use PDQ directly from the NLM's central computer through commercial time-sharing networks using most telephone modem/microcomputer or computer terminal equipment hookups. This enables clinicians to access PDQ in their homes or offices. PDQ is also available to individual users from two commercial on-line information system

This article was originally presented to the Eastern Communication Association Conference in Syracuse, New York on May, 1987.

vendor delivery systems in the United States, BRS/Saunders, as part of their COLLEAGUE information system, and from Mead Data Central, as well as in Europe through the Foundation Suisse Telemed delivery system.

Development of the PDQ Information System

The National Cancer Act of 1971 provided the NCI with the authority and mandate to develop and operate national networks to disseminate current information about cancer prevention, diagnosis, and treatment to physicians, other health professionals, and to the general public (DeVita, 1983). NCI's International Cancer Research Data Bank (ICRDB) was established as a result of the National Cancer Act. Initially, the ICRDB created computerized catalogs of information about cancer research for dissemination primarily to cancer research investigators, which ultimately led to the development of the PDQ information system.

In 1976 a new file, CLINPROT, was added to the ICRDB computer catalogs to list research protocols sponsored by the NCI. The treatment protocols in the CLINPROT file were organized generally by cancer type, but were not organized by specific cancer stages, subtypes, or geographical location. Thus, while CLINPROT provided information about current and completed studies, it offered physicians little help in identifying specific protocols relevant to their cancer patients' individual situations (NCI, 1983). PDQ was developed to improve the applicability of clinical research data available via CLINPROT by geographically matrixing protocols (those supported by the NCI and hundreds of others submitted by health care institutions as a result of ongoing NCI solicitations for submissions) and their participating investigators, as well as listing protocols by cancer stage and subtype, so physicians could obtain information on investigators and institutions in any geographic location that are (or have been) conducting studies on the type of cancer in which the searching physician was interested. Information on the database is updated monthly to provide users with the most current research available. PDQ, by providing physicians with accessible, up-to-date information about the prognosis and treatment of cancer, is designed to enable the NCI to improve cancer prevention, cancer treatment, and extend the nation's capacity to reduce cancer mortality.

Organization of the PDQ Information System

The PDQ database consists of three component files: 1) a cancer information and treatment file; 2) a file of ongoing treatment protocols; and 3) a directory file of physicians and organizations that provide cancer care. These three files are internally linked to enable highly interactive searching and retrieval of information by users of the system. The cancer information and treatment file contains prognostic and clinical information about more than 80 major cancers (NCI, 1984). A general summary (capsule statement) and a detailed summary (state-of-the-art statement) are provided for each type of cancer. Each detailed summary provides current information on prognosis, relevant staging and cellular classification systems, and a description of comparable treatment options considered to be "state-of-the-art" treatment by type and/or stage of disease. Key citations from the medical literature are provided for the user to review. When there is no effective treatment for a particular type or stage of cancer, a description of the investigational approaches that are currently under evaluation in clinical research trials is provided. The cancer information file provides a convenient point of entry into the protocol and directory files, where system users can identify specific research studies being conducted and clinicians studying the type of cancer in which they are interested. Additionally, the protocol and directory files can be searched by the specific geographic area identified by the user.

The protocol file contains summaries of more than 1,000 active treatment protocols directly supported by the NCI or submitted for inclusion in PDQ by clinical investigators throughout the world. Each protocol summary provides study objectives, patient entry criteria, details of the treatment regimen, special study parameters, and information about who is performing the trial and where it is being conducted.

The directory file contains the names, addresses, and telephone numbers of more than 10,000 physicians who devote a major portion of their clinical practice to the treatment of cancer patients, as well as a list of approximately 2,000 health care institutions where cancer research and treatment is performed. The physician listings in the directory file are composed of a compilation of the membership directories of 13 cancer-related professional societies, as well as of physicians who have applied for inclusion in the directory file. The institutional listings in the directory include organizations affiliated with the American Association of Cancer Institutes, the Association of Community Cancer Centers, cancer treatment centers funded by the NCI and their affiliates, and organizations with hospital cancer programs approved by the American College of Surgeons' Commission on Cancer.

The prognostic and treatment information contained in the cancer information file was developed and refined with the assistance of over 400 cancer specialists who served as reviewers and medical consultants. A two-tiered Editorial Board which is composed of 72 prominent medical, surgical, pediatric, and radiation oncologists has been established to maintain the currency and accuracy of the medical information in PDQ and to modify the content of the summaries based on new data (Culliton, 1985). A core group of this editorial board meets monthly at the NCI to peer-review new data as they develop, evaluate on-line data, and update information in the PDQ information files.

The Role of Information in Cancer Care

Health care providers depend on a variety of communication media such as books, journals, professional conferences, and seminars to help them learn about the latest techniques for diagnosing and treating health problems. Yet, since health care information and technologies are expanding at such a rapid rate and the numbers of medical publications and meetings are dramatically proliferating to disseminate advances in medical knowledge, it is difficult for health care providers to keep abreast of the latest relevant treatment information (Harlem, 1977; Kreps & Thornton, 1984; Day, 1975). In health care there is often a serious information and knowledge gap between the medical research community, specialized practice community, general practice community, and health care consumers (Baker, 1979; Brenner & Logan, 1980; Feldman, 1966; McIntosh, 1974). To guarantee effective treatment efforts must be taken to ensure that there is a minimal information gap between the science and research component of the medical community on the one hand, and the internist, family practitioner, patient, and general public on the other (Kreps, Ruben, Baker, & Rosenthal, 1984; Kreps, 1985; 1986).

This is especially true in the area of cancer research, where cancer treatment knowledge is expanding at an extremely rapid rate, largely due to the implementation of many concerted cancer research programs, most supported by the NCI (DeVita, 1983). Moreover, approximately 85 percent of all cancer patients are currently being treated by community physicians, who have a difficult time keeping up with the latest advances in cancer research (Culliton, 1985). As cancer treatment knowledge expands, there is an increasing need to make this new information available to those individuals who can use the data to help cancer patients and to preserve health (Siegal, 1982).

Cancer Information Diffusion and PDQ Evaluation Efforts

PDQ is only one of a number of information dissemination media employed by the NCI to promote cancer information diffusion to the cancer treatment community and general public. The Scientific Information Branch (SIB) of the NCI administers several media including computerized cancer databases (such as PDQ, CANCERLINE, CANCERLIT, CANCEREXPRESS, CANCERPROJ, and CLINPROT) and scientific journals and publications (such as *Cancer Treatment Reports, Journal of the National Cancer Institute*, the NCI Monograph series, the Cancergram series, and the Oncology Overviews series) for the dissemination of technical cancer information to scientists and physicians about the most significant recent developments in the prevention and treatment of cancer (NCI, 1984). The Office of Cancer Communication of the NCI produces and disseminates a variety of publications concerning cancer prevention and treatment and administers more than 20 regional and national Cancer Information Service (CIS) offices to provide the general public with cancer information, largely through the 1-800-4-CANCER information telephone number available nationally. Almost all of the CIS offices have direct access to PDQ and may serve an important gatekeeper function in the dissemination of PDQ information. Physicians and the general public who do not have direct access to PDQ can request PDQ information from Cancer Information Service offices.

In addition to the NCI cancer information dissemination media there are many other sources of cancer information from cancer-related professional societies and public organizations like the American Cancer Society. The variety of different cancer information dissemination vehicles available to physicians and the public complicates evaluation of the PDQ information system. "Evaluation of the impact of PDQ must account for the factor that PDQ is one of many cancer control elements influencing the cancer care system" (Sondik & Maibach, 1984, p. 368). Due to the complexity of the cancer information dissemination system and the role of PDQ in this system, PDQ evaluation efforts will be multifaceted and ongoing. Preliminary evaluation of PDQ has focused on PDQ adoption and usage trends, as well as initial reactions to PDQ by selected users.

Formative Evaluation of PDQ to Direct System Development

Currently a large scale evaluation of PDQ is being undertaken to provide key information about the use of the system and to address whether there has been diffusion of the information in the PDQ system to relevant public audiences. Such information is crucial for directing further development of PDQ as part of the NCI's cancer control efforts (Kreps, Hubbard, & DeVita, 1988). If the goal of reducing the 1980 cancer death rate in the United States by half is to be met by the year 2000, PDQ must be an effective channel for disseminating cancer information to the cancer treatment community and the general public (DeVita, 1983; Kreps & Naughton, 1986).

There are four components (A, B, C, and D) to the PDQ evaluation plan (Sondik & Maibach, 1984; Kreps, Hubbard, & DeVita, 1988). Component A of the evaluation is a comprehensive review and assessment of the processes by which the information contained within the PDQ system was collected and is maintained. Component B is an assessment of the technical characteristics and competence of the PDQ information system and the delivery systems it employs, as well as an examination of PDQ distribution and usage trends. Component C of the evaluation is an assessment of system dissemination activities and user reactions to the PDQ system to identify areas for technical revisions, potential new users, and strategies for expanding system use.

Component D of the evaluation plan is to assess the impact of the PDQ system on the diffusion of state-of-the-art cancer treatment information in the medical community and the resultant impact on cancer treatment, morbidity, and mortality. Each of the four components of the PDQ evaluation is designed to provide reflexive information to administrators of the PDQ system about current levels of performance, acceptance, and impact of PDQ. Such information will be channeled back into the PDQ system to direct system enhancements and innovations in system implementation.

Ongoing formative evaluation of the PDQ information system has helped identify key issues, problems, and stumbling blocks in the implementation of the PDQ system and in effective dissemination of cancer information (Kreps & Naughton, 1986). Evaluation data were gathered about levels of use of the PDQ system and about users' reactions to the performance of the system (see the following for examples PDQ evaluation data: Kreps, Hubbard, & DeVita, 1988; Kreps, Maibach, Naughton, Day, & Annett, 1986; Kreps & Naughton, 1986). These data helped identify performance gaps between actual system use and optimal system use, and helped to increase the reflexivity of the National Cancer Institute by providing PDQ administrators with information about specific communication problems and needs of PDQ users. For example, evaluation research data provided PDQ administrators with information about potential new information sources, new audiences, new delivery media, and innovations for the PDQ system for enhancing health information dissemination efforts for the future. A key lesson learned from the PDQ evaluation is that to effectively disseminate health information to relevant audiences, organizations must be able to gather reflexive data about system performance and use these data to guide information dissemination strategies and delivery system innovations to meet the needs of system users (Kreps, 1988). Continued formative evaluation and refinement of the PDQ system can facilitate effective dissemination of relevant cancer treatment information to those individuals that need such information and enhance the quality of cancer care.

References

Baker, S. 1979. The diffusion of high technology medical innovation: the computed tomography scanner example. *Social Science and Medicine* 13, 155-62.

Brenner, D. and Logan, R. 1980. Some considerations in the diffusion of medical technologies: Medical information systems. In D. Nimmo (ed.), *Communication Yearbook* 4. New Brunswick, NJ: Transaction-International Communication Association, 609-23.

Covell, D. C., Uman, G. C., and Manning, P. R. 1985. Information needs in office practice: Are they being met? *Annals of Internal Medicine* 103, 596-99.

Culliton, B. J. 1985. Information as a "cure" for cancer. *Science*, 227, p. 732.

Day, S. 1975. *Communication of scientific information*. Paris: S. Karger.

DeVita, V. T., Jr. 1985. Cancer as a preventable disease. *Maryland Medical Journal* 34, 41-43.

DeVita, V. T. 1983, September. PDQ: Bringing the latest in cancer diagnosis and treatment to the community physician. *Your Patient and Cancer*, 88-45.

Harlem, O. 1977. *Communication in medicine.* Paris: S. Karger.

Feldman, J. 1966. *The dissemination of health information.* Chicago: Aldine.

Kreps, G. L. 1988. The pervasive role of information in health and health care: Implications for health communication policy. In J. Anderson (ed.), *Communication Yearbook* 11 (pp. 238-76), Beverly Hills, CA: Sage.

Kreps, G. L., Hubbard, S. M., and DeVita, V. T. 1988. The role of the Physician Data Query on-line cancer system in health information dissemination. In B. Ruben (ed.), *Information and Behavior 2* (pp. 362-74), New Brunswick, NJ: Transaction Press.

Kreps, G. L., Maibach, E. W., Naughton, M. D., Day, S. H., and Annett, D. Q. 1986. PDQ usage trends: Implications for evaluation. In A. Levy and B. Williams (eds.), *Proceedings of the American Association for Medical Systems and Informatics Congress 86.* Washington, DC: AAMSI, 71-75.

Kreps, G. L. and Naughton, M. D. 1986. The role of PDQ in disseminating cancer information. In R. Salaman, B. Blum, and M. Jorgensen (eds.), *MEDINFO 1986.* Amsterdam: North Holland Press/Elsevier Science Publishers, 400-404.

Kreps, G. L., Ruben, B. D., Baker, M. W., and Rosenthal, S. R. 1987. A national survey of public knowledge about digestive health and diseases. *Public Health Reports,* 102, 270-77.

Kreps, G. L. and Thornton, B. C. 1984. *Health communication: Theory and practice.* New York: Longman Inc.

McIntosh, J. 1974. Process of communication, information seeking control associated with cancer: a selected review of the literature. *Social Science and Medicine 8,* 167-87.

NCI. 1984. *A guide to scientific information services of the National Cancer Institute.* U.S. Department of Health and Human Services, NIH Publication No. 84-2683.

NCI. 1983. *PDQ: A new computerized database for physicians treating cancer patients.* Unpublished in-house report of the National Cancer Institute.

Penniman, W. D., Dominick, W. E. 1980. Monitoring and evaluation of on-line information system usage. *Information Processing and Management 116,* 17-35.

Rice, R. E., Borgman, C. L. 1983. The use of computer-monitored data in information science and communication research. *Journal of the American Society for Information Science 34,* 247-56.

Siegel, E. R. 1982. Transfer of information to health practitioners. In B. Dervin, and M. Voight (eds.), *Progress in Communication Sciences,* Vol. III. Norwood, NJ: Ablex.

Sondik, E. J. and Maibach, E. W. 1984. PDQ evaluation. *Proceedings of the 8th Annual Symposium on Computer Applications in Medical Care,* 368-71.

Webb, E., Campbell, D., Schwartz, R., and Sechrist, L. 1966. *Unobtrusive measures: Nonreactive research in the social sciences.* Chicago: Rand McNally.

CHAPTER
7

Culture and Health Communication

Culture has a pervasive influence on health and health care. We are all acculturated by our diverse cultural affiliations through repetitive reinforcing metacommunicative processes that socialize us to accept specific culturally-approved (normative) health beliefs and engage in culturally-approved health behaviors. Our cultural influences are many; they can be based on national origin, ethnic background, race, religion, regional affiliation, gender, age, education, socio-economic status, professional and occupational status, sexual orientation, health status, disabilities, and a host of other social factors. There are many differences among these cultures in the norms established for health and health care, making the provision of health care in our modern multicultural society very complex and challenging.

Cultural socialization processes are often very powerful. It is not uncommon for members of one cultural group to become ethnocentric (believing that their cultural orientation is the only legitimate perspective) about their health beliefs. Ethnocentric attitudes toward health care often complicate health care delivery, leading to stereotyping of and prejudicial treatment toward people who do not hold similar cultural orientations. It is not uncommon in modern health care for a consumer to have his or her health beliefs questioned and even violated. Violation of cultural norms is not tolerated easily and leads to distrust, frustration, and hostility. Health care providers and consumers must communicate carefully and sensitively with one another to recognize and demonstrate respect for cultural differences. Awareness of culturally related terminology, beliefs, values, and attitudes is a requirement for modern health care practice (Kreps & Thornton, 1992). This section of the book examines many issues concerning cultural sensitivity and effective cross-cultural communication in health care.

The first reading in this chapter, "Destroyers and Healers," written by Patrick Cooke, first appeared in the magazine *In Health* which addresses health care for native American Indians in Montana. Minority groups in the United States, whether American Indian, African American, Asian American or Hispanic, often contend that their health care needs are not adequately met. This reading clearly illustrates the many problems faced by both clients and providers at the Indian Health Service. The author notes how the differences in tribes, the difficulty of providing services, the lack of funding, and the health care bureaucracy conspire to complicate health care for native Americans. It is clear, however, that the pervading issue is culture. The Indians and the health care providers have two colliding cultural perspectives on health care. After reading this article, reflect not only on the problems of the American Indian, but also on African Americans living in Harlem, abused women who are single heads of family, the homeless, the indigent aged, and the many Hispanic people who face similar health care problems. The difficulties inherent in providing the best quality health care to diverse cultural groups must not be underestimated.

The second reading, "Cross-cultural Concerns and Communication in Health Care" by Dorothy Rasinski (who is both a physician and a lawyer), identifies key questions and patterns of treatment health care providers should be aware of when interacting with clients of cultures other than their own. This reading stresses the importance of communicating sensitively not only with the client, but also with the client's family and support network. The author contends that health care providers need a clear understanding of their clients' cultural background and orientations to their health problems and health care treatment. After reading this article, review the Values History at the end of the reading. This is an important document used to determine the beliefs, values, and attitudes of clients so treatment can be geared to the individual. Try answering some of the Values History questions yourself.

Kreps, G. L. & Thornton, B. C. (1992). *Health Communication: Theory and Practice* 2nd edition. Prospect Heights, IL: Waveland Press.

15

Destroyers and Healers

By Patrick Cooke

Young George Reed flew a hundred feet through the air the night he wrecked his sister's pickup on the Crow Indian reservation road between Prior and Saint Xavier. Accidents happen on empty and unreal highways like this in southern Montana. The Indians who travel it talk of how moonlight on the land and a curved sky full of stars will veer the mind in funny ways.

For a long time George lay there in the April wind beneath the Bighorn Mountains until at last an ambulance rode out the forty-some miles from Billings and raced him back into town. People were pretty amazed when, a week later, George walked out of the hospital. In a couple of months he was cowboyin' again on ranches up north and went on to work the Montana Centennial Cattle Drive. Young George had a lot of kick in him at 24 years old, so no one expected he would be dead nine months after the smashup.

"We buried him a week ago." George's father, George Reed, Jr., speaks in the slow, gutteral cadences the bilingual Crow Indians bring to English. "He died at the Indian Health Service hospital of improper care." Like many men of the tribe, the elder George is tall and as hard as an iron bar, but he has the dazed, exhausted look of a hostage. "The doctors told us my son died of the DTs, but I know he didn't."

The father remembers that it was about December when his son began complaining of gut pains, that young George went to the Indian Health Service hospital on the Crow reservation and that there they gave him an antacid and sent him home. Three more times during the month he went back to the reservation hospital, each time feeling worse. He was finally admitted in January, and a blood test revealed trouble with his pancreas. He was treated for ulcers and the DTs, the often fatal delirium and tremors that come from drinking too much, too long. All of young George's complaints, in fact, were consistent with hard drinking. His father doesn't deny that his son might have taken a drink

Reprinted with permission from In Health 22 (1990:66-76). Mr. Cooke is a contributing editor to In Health magazine.

or two in the weeks leading up to his death, but the cowboys young George had been riding with swear that he hadn't been on any bender. "He'd been out on the ranch, and like any other normal American citizen you got to go to a bar and socialize a bit afterward, that's all," says the older George. No, the father insists, it was something from that car wreck catching up with young George, but whatever it was, the Indian Health Service doctors didn't pick it up.

"It was just after midnight that he stood up and gagged and gasped for air," the father says of his son's final moments last January in the reservation hospital. "He recognized me, he knew who I was. But he was in so much pain he was tearing down the curtains. We were yelling that they should do something for him but the doctor on duty said, 'This is just withdrawal that comes with the DTs.' Then George fell over backwards. My wife screamed and another doctor came running in, but my son was dead by then."

That young George would die was unforeseen, but unremarkable. For the one and a half million Native Americans born into more than 800 tribes in the U.S. mainland and Alaska, the chances of dying begin early: Between ages one and four, the risk is more than twice what it is for other American children. Between the ages of 25 and 34 the chances are roughly three times as high. Murder and suicide occur about twice as often on the reservation — the rez, as it's called — and fatal accidents are three times more common. Indians die with greater frequency of pneumonia, influenza, infections, tuberculosis, diabetes, and alcoholic cirrhosis, which occurs 18 times more often than in the general population. Young George was tough, but he couldn't buck his chances: As an Indian it was three times more likely that he would die before he reached age 45 than if he had been born a non-Indian. Those are just the odds in Indian country.

It's easy to blame those odds on continued neglect from white America. And many Indians do. The United States government first promised to provide health care free of charge for American Indians in the 19th century, when treaties stipulated that it would come as part of an exchange for lands. But until 1955, when the Indian Health Service was established, treatment was, as one might guess, perfunctory. And since then, health care has fluctuated between dismal and respectable. The fact is, however, that the Indian Health Service, a part of the Department of Health and Human Services, has an absurd task that's roughly the equivalent of running a Third-World relief effort on a shoestring budget. For 35 years the agency has been tap dancing between charges of neglect if it fails in its job, and paternalism if it succeeds.

No two tribes are alike, which means the service must accommodate dozens of languages and tribal hierarchies. Its clinics and hospitals serve far-flung rural folk as well as urban dwellers plagued by drugs and city stresses. The steadily growing Indian population and intermarriage outside the reservation mean that more Indians must be cared for by roughly the same number of dollars. Distances are often so vast that health care arrives only by plane or helicopter.

If private industry had been administering Indian health care it would have
gotten out of the business decades ago.

The Crow reservation where young George grew up is part of the Indian
Health Service's "Billings Area" — there are 11 such Areas nationwide — which
serves 50,000 Indians on eight reservations in Montana and Wyoming. There
are, among others, Blackfeet, Cheyenne, Crow, Shoshone, Sioux, Salish,
Arapahoe, Gros Ventre, and Chippewa-Cree. Of the 45 doctors who work the
three hospitals and a number of small clinics scattered throughout the area,
only two are Indian. Most are white — "Anglos." It is one of Indian country's
abundant ironies that because they are white and doctors, they are the
conflicting symbols of both the destroyer who diminished Indians to reservation
life and the healer who now safeguards their well-being there.

"It's always been a power struggle between the Indian Health Service and
the tribe." The Crow health director, paid by the tribe to convey its concerns
to the health service's local administrators, is a friendly but disconsolate-looking
Crow named — honest — Quentin Big Medicine. "They're just bureaucrats with
secure jobs down at the hospital; they put in their years and then retire. Go
down there and speak to them. They'll come up with a lot of statistics for you,
but it's just talk. They've never cared about us. We don't even get real doctors
here. All we get are interns."

What happened to young George Reed is typical of the heartless treatment
at the hospital — wrong prescriptions, incorrect diagnoses, disregarded
complaints — say some of the Crow who use its services. Crow men such as
Cornelius Little Light grunt at the mention of the place. Floyd Real Bird laughs
and walks away. "There's no courtesy, no human warmth with those people,"
is what Phillip Beaumont, Sr., says. "They look at you as an Indian and you
get the bum's rush — write that down!"

"We were all standing there when my son died," the elder George says in
a hollow voice. "After they pronounced him dead my son's girlfriend just started
beating the shit out of the doctor. 'You killed him! You killed him!' she was
screaming."

That's the kind of thing the Crow are driven to, says the father. "That's what
you've got to do. You've got to push people up against the wall to get your
way. Otherwise, they look at you and they think you're nothin', just a dumb
son-of-a-bitch."

More than a hundred years ago, the scraps of George Custer's 7th Cavalry
were slung into a mass grave atop Last Stand Hill on what is now the Crow
reservation. It was the cavalry's Crow scouts who reluctantly guided Custer
into the Little Bighorn Valley, sensibly wailing their death chants as they rode,
and tribes such as the Sioux and Cheyenne who put an end to the general.

The battlefield's Stars and Stripes snap in a cold sky now where hawks circle
out over the prairie below, over the small Crow village, the decaying rodeo
grandstands, and the abandoned Sun Lodge Motel with its busted windows
and tumbleweed-blown swimming pool. Farther on are other failed Indian

businesses, like the electronics factory and the carpet mill; the Crow Revival Center has the look of a bomb-damaged building. So many dreams of a better future in this valley steal away on the magnificent wind.

Young George Reed died in the 34-bed reservation hospital that the U.S. government built in 1930 down by the Little Bighorn River. It is the busiest place in the Crow village. There is a dental office, a pharmacy, an optometrist's office, alcohol and diabetes treatment centers, and a weight-training room. Anglo doctors stroll the halls with bright Indian beading woven around their stethoscopes. The hospital is down at the heels in places, but it is doubtful there is a similar town in rural America — roughly 6,000 patients are served and the unemployment rate is about 60 percent — that can boast it has it this good.

"You can see what we've built here over time," says Jim Upchurch, tipping back in his chair in a small room away from the rush of the hospital corridors. Upchurch, a good-natured Anglo and one of ten doctors on the reservation, is the chief medical officer at the hospital and well acquainted with the events of the night young George died.

Upchurch came to the Crow reservation five years ago as part of the National Health Service Corps, a now moribund federal program that paid medical school bills in exchange for time spent in places where it was hard to get physicians to practice, such as inner cities and country towns. When Upchurch's obligation was completed he stayed on. At one time, reservations were often these doctors' first postings, and thus was born the sarcastic tag "intern" among the tribes for *any* Indian Health Service doctor.

When the captive work force diminished, *every* Area became responsible for its own recruiting. The Billings Area office has a full-time recruiter who spends a great deal of time extolling the wonders of the wide open spaces to doctors. He's had limited success. Until recently, the Crow reservation hospital had been three doctors short for several years, and in order to keep the doctors they *do* have they must pay something close to parity with rural doctors' salaries outside — around $55,000 to start.

Paying doctors well, and covering their malpractice liability, cuts into Area budgets. And the budgets haven't kept up with medical costs. In 1987, for example, the service had $845 to spend per person; the rest of the nation spent $1,987 per person for health care. Something had to give, and it has: The Office of Technology Assessment in Washington, D.C., estimated that in 1988 alone 28,000 elective procedures for Indian patients were postponed. In the Billings Area, many were potentially lifesaving services: obstetrical exams, mammograms, and psychiatric care for suicidal teenagers. "The IHS was rationing long before the rest of the country," says Duane Jeanotte, a taciturn North Dakota Chippewa who is the head of the Billings Area. "It's hard when someone comes to you and says, 'Why can't you take care of my daughter's knee problems?' How do you tell them you don't have the money?"

As a result, according to the 1988 study, the service spends nearly $90 million of its $1 billion budget on acute care: imminent, emergency room situations such as auto accidents, fights, and domestic brawls. Jeanotte estimates that the Billings Area spends from 40 to 60 percent of its budget on alcohol-related injuries and illnesses. Washington, D.C., mindful of the public eye, pressures for prevention programs to stop alcoholism before it causes accidents, for example, but the physicians on the reservation haven't the time, money, or staff.

It's a shame that all this should have happened, because prior to the budget crunch, the Indian Health Service was slowly achieving victories nationwide against long-entrenched health problems. Maternal mortality, for example, was once twice as high in Indian country as for the general U.S. population; now it is roughly equal. Infant mortality (birth through 28 days) is now actually lower on the reservation than for the rest of the nation. Fetal alcohol syndrome has dropped by more than half in the Billings Area over the past ten years, as it has on many reservations. Ambulance service has improved, and better sanitation is curbing gastrointestinal diseases.

The Indian Health Service charter states only that it shall "elevate Indian health to the highest possible level." For better or worse, the slightly rundown Crow hospital beside the river is a working translation of that mandate. That's why the staff felt gratified last year when a survey of patients harvested comments like "Excellent doctors!" "The nurses are always courteous!" "Keep up the good work!"

"I can show you hundreds of people who say the care is good here," says Upchurch, who received the rare honor of being adopted by the tribe two years ago. "They are people who wouldn't go anywhere else." Like many physicians who work in Indian health, he is frequently protective of the tribe, even when village grumbling demonstrates the feeling isn't always reciprocated.

But what of those voices in the village, the ones who charge that no one cares about Indians? What about the people who look at the numbers of Indians dying and don't wonder that young George Reed became one of them?

"We provide good care here," Upchurch says in response to the routine criticisms. "Every doctor, every day of the year.

"Sure, I know they call us interns," he says, "but every doctor here is board certified and every one is here because they *want* to be." In fact, he insists, many feel far closer in spirit to the tribes they serve than to the federal agency in Washington, D.C., that they work for.

"I really can't discuss the George Reed case," Upchurch says. "But, you know, this really pisses me off." He is suddenly fuming after hearing the older George's version of that January night's events. "I mean, we get blamed for a lot of people's self-destructive behavior here. Well, the fact is I can't say anything. I'd *love* to, I really would."

Upchurch quickly dials a nearby telephone and asks the hospital's director if he may talk about the case. He is told that he may not. The release of medical information within the government services is almost unheard of. For a long moment, Upchurch sits shaking his head trying to compose himself. "This is the kind of thing that will chase doctors away, accusations that we don't care," he says calmly now, but with blood still in his eye. "Hell, if I didn't care would I work in a place that's sixty years old and put up with some of the things we put up with? Man, this is just making my day."

Ninety-seven percent of the land Indians once claimed has been lost to the white man. By the time manifest destiny completed the long push west, it had left in its wake an Indian race crushed by disease, starvation, massacre, and, finally, neglect. Generations of whites assumed, if they gave the matter any thought at all, that those Indians hardy enough to survive the trampling would surrender the old ways and dissolve into the melting pot. Certainly some have, but the idea of wholesale assimilation does not sit well with most Indians.

Segregation, however, has its price. Inner voices send conflicting messages: Protect what is Indian and abhor what is white, demands one voice; the other whispers that the only escape from a cycle of isolation and poverty is to live the white's way. The effects of racial identity on well-being may be impossible to measure, but no one denies that depression, alcoholism, and suicide are what come of hearing voices.

"I once saw a sign in Sheridan, Wyoming, that said No Dogs or Indians Allowed — and we didn't even get top billing," says Dale Old Horn, an outspoken Crow and a Massachusetts Institute of Technology graduate who insists that not only past insults but current white racism affect the health and welfare of many tribes. "I'm not talking about a hundred years ago. I saw this in my lifetime. Are things getting better in 1990 for Indians? I don't see chronic alcoholism and child abuse in Indian America as improved conditions."

Passing through the doors of the chalet-styled Indian Health Service clinic on the Northern Cheyenne reservation at Lame Deer, 45 miles east of the Crow hospital, means crossing from one world into another, passing from Indian time into white man's time. Outside, wounded-looking teenagers glide slowly by in pickup trucks, and skittish village dogs hobble among houses and rusted trailers. Inside, four Anglo doctors attend to a silent tableau of expressionless Cheyenne awaiting their turn in a reception room booming with the noise of "Flintstones" cartoons on TV.

Dave Means is the clinic's gentle-mannered administrator, but more importantly he is the liaison between the Cheyenne in the reception area and the Indian Health Service Anglos. Although he is Sioux, Means grew up amid the Cheyenne's tall pines and high country around Lame Deer. Because the Indian Health Service signs his paycheck, some Indians have accused him of turning "apple," as red-on-the-outside-white-on-the-inside defectors are called.

But the slur hardly seems fair. Means, after all, remembers well when the white doctor showed up only three days a week in Lame Deer, and how his own father had to hold on for 48 hours after a heart attack because he happened to be stricken on the wrong day. He knows, too, the "Lysol houses," rooms where some Indians go to still the voices by mixing batches of "Montana gin," a cocktail produced by poking a hole in a can of disinfectant or hair spray and mixing the alcohol inside with orange soda. Dave Means knows all about growing up Indian and feeling lost, a creature of neither the white nor red worlds. "We were raised to believe that white is bad," says Means, speaking in the subdued tones common to everyone in Lame Deer. "So to be 'good' for us immediately meant being the opposite, an outsider in white America. But if we were good and they were bad, how come they had things we couldn't have, like liquor? The rez is 'dry,' so when I would come back from drinking I'd feel like a criminal. And when you feel like a criminal you think, 'I'm not going to have just one beer, I'm going to drink a whole six-pack.' That's how confused you are.

"An Indian may say something to a white man — an insult or even a compliment — that will completely pass the white by," he says of the doctors and Indian Health Service officials who come through Lame Deer. "It will make perfect sense to me. But if you work here as a white you constantly risk misunderstanding or being misunderstood.

"For whites there are specific times to do things that Indians are required to adapt to here at the clinic, like appointments," says Means. "But for the Indian, time has a different meaning: The forest is there, the rocks are there, the earth lives.

"Indians also tend to talk around a matter rather than directly about it, which drives whites crazy. I'll give you an example: A doctor will ask, 'When did these symptoms start?' expecting to hear the events of the last few days or weeks. But the Indian says, '1968,' and goes on to communicate in a series of long stories, which is the Indian way of communicating. The problem is that the doctor can see out the door that he has fifteen patients waiting. 'Then in 1974 . . .' the Indian goes on with another story, and the doctor is thinking: 'Get to the point.' A lot of times if an Indian feels the doctor is impatient he'll just walk out believing no one cares to take the time. So the medicine must be no good. The most popular doctors here have been the ones who are slowest and least popular with their peers, who then have to pick up the slack."

As an Anglo doctor at the Lame Deer clinic, Jon Hauxwell walks as fine a line as Dave Means does as an Indian. Thirteen years ago Hauxwell left Kansas City, Kansas, for the Cheyenne clinic because, he says, "I didn't want to be just another doc in a medical arts building someplace." In that time he has lost his need for a cultural translator and has seen care improve at the Cheyenne reservation. But he's also seen perhaps 15 doctors come and go, some because of cabin fever, others because they never understood the special conflicts that sicken their patients.

"You have to have some sense of what happened to these people and the obliteration of their culture." says Hauxwell, who has been invited to dance with the exclusive Gourd Dance Society at powwows and to partake in "giveaways," ceremonial events in which impoverished Cheyenne hand out imprudently lavish gifts. "Their medicine and spirit life were nearly annihilated quite casually by white technology. What does that do to your ability to see the future? Even today it's still the cause of insecurity and self-doubt."

From the bountiful nation beyond the reservation, it is tempting to dismiss poor health and Indian despair as a character defect or the failing of a people to get a grip on themselves; but then Calvinist-inspired Anglos have long judged the world by the virtues of abstinence, clean living, and industry. Here, beside the slow, gray road that passes through Lame Deer on its journey out of Montana, those Anglo virtues seem distant luxuries.

Exiles of a sort are what Means and Hauxwell see passing through the doors of the clinic, withdrawn and out of choices, strung out on the white man's liquor and dying on the worst of the white man's diet. The clinic cannot still the voices, or reverse history, or drag people into the light of good health if they feel no need to come. All the clinic can do is try to ease the strain and search for larger signs of hope.

Sometimes the signs come. Last New Year's Eve, the town of Lame Deer held a sobriety dance. Five hundred people showed up, a turnout that would have been unimaginable a few years ago. "I think some people are beginning to say, 'I've had enough of this booze,'" says Dave Means. "'The tribe has had enough.'"

Still, change arrives slowly here, no matter whose time it's measured on. "You know, we never saw obese people on the reservation years ago," says Means, lamenting his diabetes-prone Indian patients. "Now? Look around you. It's ironic — for so many years the problem was not having enough to eat. Now it's junk food."

He might have said: The whites once starved us, then they threw us crumbs. Now Washington sends money to fight obesity, but they also send surplus butter and cheese.

Not long after the battle of the Little Bighorn, the majestic Sioux chief Gall, who was suspected of actually killing Custer, traveled to Washington, D.C. The government gave the chief money to spend, but upon finding beggars in the city where the Great Father lived, he gave it all away.

There are still beggars in the Great Father's city, and 114 years after the Little Bighorn, still debates about what to do with his native children. It is an unbreakable circle: Indians such as Quentin Big Medicine and George Reed, Jr., do not trust the doctors on the reservation. The doctors so doubt the wisdom of the Indian Health Service in Washington, D.C. that they call it "Disneyland East." The Indian Health Service has little confidence that Congress can be sensitive to its growing needs. And, alas, Congress says it is as penniless as Gall.

Last summer a special Senate committee ended a two-year investigation that again looked into Indian matters — America's first federal investigation ever, in 1792, dealt with Indians. What the latest probe found in the Bureau of Indian Affairs and the Indian Health Service were the kinds of swindles that have become commonplace in Indian country: waste, abuse, fraud.

For example, in Minnesota's Bemidji Area, according to the committee, Indian Health Service officials treated themselves and friends to money earmarked for Indian medical care and health education, threatening to fire employees who reported irregularities. In New Mexico, Area administrators forged signatures on documents, paid kickbacks, and squandered government money on travel. The Senate committee claims that the Indian Health Service knew of much of the waste and corruption, and not only silenced an internal investigation, but also ignored the Inspector General's Office recommendations that might have saved the health service $37 million. In fact, in 1989, two independent management firms hired by the service itself reported that their client had earned the reputation of being "without question, the most poorly managed of all the agencies in the Department of Health and Human Services."

One item that particularly steamed senators was a retreat the Indian Health Service sponsored two years ago at a resort called Sunrise Springs, near Santa Fe, New Mexico. The week-long program was designed in part to instruct tribal leaders from the Albuquerque Area on the benefits of fitness and a healthy lifestyle. Those leaders were then expected to return to their tribes and institute health programs on the reservations — a kind of "trickle down" therapy.

The event, however, was poorly attended by those who would benefit most; only two tribal representatives showed up. "Most of the other three dozen participants," the committee report states, "were managers from the Indian Health Service Headquarters [in Washington, D.C.] or the Albuquerque Area Office." This gathering underwent such dubious treatments as massage therapy, acupuncture, and "alpha chamber wellness services for stress reduction." Investigators wondered how the satin warm-up jackets, visors, and bumper stickers given to participants to commemorate their stay served poverty-stricken Indians back on the reservation. The $70,000 excursion was paid for, says the committee, with congressional funds intended for the Indian Juvenile Alcohol and Drug Abuse Prevention Program.

"I sanctioned the retreat and I still don't have any problem with the concept," says Craig Vanderwagen, the director of health promotion programs for the Indian Health Service. Vanderwagen is a tall, soft-talking Anglo who grew up on the Zuni reservation in New Mexico and later worked there as a physician — one of his patients was the tribal governor, who died of alcoholism. Now he spends much of his time in an office building that looks out over mirrored high-rises reflecting the mega-malls and fast food joints of a depressing Washington suburb. Vanderwagen has been told not to discuss Sunrise Springs, presumably by the same bureaucratic hierarchy that the congressional investigation found to be "significantly uncooperative," but his frontier independence overrules.

"Why is it that when private industry puts on a retreat like this in order to build leadership, that's considered brilliant; but when government does the same thing it's regarded as a waster of taxpayers' money?" he asks. "I'll tell you what's going to happen five years down the road when somebody says, 'Why don't you *do* something about these terrible problems?' *Nobody* is going to take the risk again to try something new. You take a risk in government and you land on the front page of the *Washington Post.*"

If the exasperated Senate has its way, incidents like Sunrise Springs will no longer be an issue. In December, the Senate committee recommended that the Indian Health Service and the Bureau of Indian Affairs be phased out altogether. Under a move being called New Federalism, all money and responsibility would be funneled directly to the tribes. At the Crow and Cheyenne reservations the new plan would mean operating like any ordinary town in Montana: They would find and hire their own doctors, build their own facilities, look after their own treatment programs. For the first time in decades, the prospect of more fraud and broken promises from whites would vanish because all accountability would fall to the tribes. If anybody got fleeced there would be no need to look beyond the reservation for the culprit.

The Indian Health Service has already encouraged some tribes to begin staffing and managing their own facilities — seven out of 50 hospitals in the past ten years. Proudly displayed on a coffee table in Vanderwagen's office is a handsome book printed by the Warm Springs Indians of Oregon, detailing the workings of their tribal-run hospital and health programs. Vanderwagen's former reservation at Zuni is doing well, too, and the tribe now operates a nationally recognized wellness center.

These are, of course, exceptions. Full Indian self-sufficiency will take time. If the busted business ventures strewn across the Little Bighorn Valley at the Crow reservation are any measure, not every tribe is ready to assume control.

And even business savvy may not assure success in a culture that views caring as more than the whites' dollars and cents. "These Indians are extremely generous people," says Toby Lantz, one of the few Anglo women living at the Cheyenne reservation. "If a family member is short of money you are *obligated* to help. People give away pots and pans full of food, Pendleton blankets, horses. If you have a job, people may be lined up outside your house on payday with their hands out. It's not a loan, it's a gift."

Despite such barriers, the notion of tribal sovereignty seems a risk worth chasing, even if it lands the Great Father in the newspaper again. Budgets are not likely to get better and there will no doubt be charges of white abandonment from some Indians. But the alternatives are continued resentment, further investigations. And more of what George Reed, Jr., convinced that agents of a distant, unmerciful government killed his son, has in store.

"I'm going to sue those sons of bitches at the hospital," he says darkly through his grief. "It won't bring my son back but maybe it'll help the Crow tribe if I put those people in their place."

Nobody has filed any lawsuits yet. It wouldn't seem right. They only just buried young George, a Crow Indian that the *Big Horn County News* wrote was a good boy from the reservation who died of "natural causes."

16

Cross-Cultural Concerns and Communication in Health Care

By *Dorothy C. Rasinski*

Introduction

Over the past several years, there has been a dramatic influx of immigrants into the United States, particularly from Central America and Southeast Asia, and including dissidents seeking political refuge. Identification with the culture of origin is frequently stronger among these groups than it is among those who were born in the United States of immigrant parents or those who immigrated earlier and have assimilated or adapted their own cultures over time. Many of these new residents find it difficult to understand what we do, how we do it, or why, in terms of health care delivery priorities and the roles of provider and patient in reaching decisions. This is particularly true where the provider and the patient (or the patient's family) come from different cultural backgrounds and have little or no awareness of the other's culture or background. Similarly, when both the provider and the patient (or patient's family) are of the same cultural background but the community in which they find themselves is different, with little familiarity with their culture, concerns may be raised on the part of other members of the health care team (particularly hospital staff and nurses) who perceive that the patient's autonomy, liberty, or freedom of choice is being restricted or infringed upon inappropriately.

Nowhere are these problems of greater importance than where they relate to issues at the beginning and the end of life, in terms of procreation, in relationships of parents to their minor children, and in the setting of terminal care and withdrawal or withholding of life-sustaining treatment. These seem

An earlier version of this paper originally appeared in *HEC* (Hospital Ethics Committee) *Forum* and was geared toward members of Ethics Committeees, (Vol. 1, p. 137, 1989). In view of its applicability to all health care providers, it has been modified by one of the original authors to apply to anyone in the health field as well as those studying to become members of the health care team. Dr. Rasinski is a physician-attorney consulting in legal medicine, bioethics and risk management.

to be among the most troublesome issues facing health care professionals today. Those involved or planning to enter these health occupations should become familiar with these potential problems, lower their own thresholds of sensitivity and awareness and assure themselves that cross-cultural concerns are being considered. The influence of the patient's ethnic background, religion, and/or lifestyle upon choices must be respected. Only then can "best interest" decisions about "quality of life" be appreciated and implemented.

I. Critical Factors to be Aware of and Questions to Raise about the Patient and his Family

The background of the patient as well as the patient's surrogate decision-maker, other family members, the physician, other health care providers or members of the health care delivery team, the facility itself, and the local community are important elements in this context. It is critical that another person, whether relative, health care provider or some other individual, not be permitted to overwhelm the patient or interfere with his or her ability to make choices or to relate to care-providers.

Items that may be appropriate to consider in such settings are the patient's culture, ethnic background, nationality, religion, intelligence, education, profession and/or work history, lifestyle, family composition and relationships, other interpersonal relationships and support groups, language, economic and social status, habits, customs, beliefs, values, perceptions of body language and "acceptable communications," place of birth, mental health, self-esteem, tolerance for questioning or discussion, sex or gender and cultural perceptions of those factors, and prior experience with or expectations of the health care system.

With respect to the patient's cultural background, the following questions may be asked:

A. Is wellness in that culture valued above disease or resorting to "Western" health care?

B. What is the cultural nature of "disease" as opposed to "illness" in that particular group? (Disease is here defined as the diagnosis reached by the medical professional; illness is what the patient senses is wrong; these are not typically identical).

C. Does disease have an "evil eye" connotation?

D. Has the individual previously been involved with a shaman, faith healer, curandera, partera, etc., who would affect any relationship with the current health care provider of "traditional American medicine?"

E. If given oral medications, will the patient ingest them as directed or place them in a "mummy bundle" in the corner of his room and expect an efficacious result? (After all, if the medicine is really "magic," it can work anywhere and need not be taken by the patient. This belief is held by many Native Americans.)

F. Are intramuscular or intravenous injections valued above oral medications? (The Chinese place such a value on parenteral medications.)

In terms of the patient's ethnic background, it is appropriate to raise issues concerning status in terms of the "local ethnic society as a whole." In this regard, one might ask:

A. Is the patient a member of an ethnic minority in the community?

B. How attached is the patient to his or her ethnic background, and how recently has he or she come to this community? How much does the patient still identify with the original nationality or ethnic values or customs?

C. Does he or she view being in the hospital as "turning one's back" on ethnic background or original culture?

D. Does the culture value or reinforce passive acceptance of whatever fate deals, as opposed to an aggressive attitude of "fighting back" against a disease process?

E. Are physicians or professional health care providers recognized or rejected by that group? Is a greater value placed on self-directed and/or family-initiated efforts to control or defeat disease or illness as opposed to "outside assistance" of whatever sort?

Under the heading of religion, the team might wish to ask the following questions:

A. Does the patient's religious affiliation construe health or illness as part of a "natural lottery," as the visitation of an angry or vengeful "God" or as punishment deserved for past sins?

B. Is there a religious value placed upon suffering, to earn a higher place in "heaven?" Is it something which the patient may use or offer to atone for his or her own or someone else's sins?

C. Is passive acceptance of suffering to be valued or strived for? Is disease, illness, or disability seen as the "Will of God" with a value to be placed on resignation to that fate?

D. How thoroughly trained is the patient in religion and are his or her practices in conformity with its dictates? Has the patient been consistent and diligent in religious practices or resumed them only recently in response to the current illness?

E. Has he or she consulted a spiritual advisor, counselor, priest, pastor, rabbi, other practitioner, medicine man, etc? If so, how recently?

F. How much family support has been provided in maintaining the liturgy or customs of the particular religion?

G. Are there "sacramental provisions" available within that religious community? Has the patient taken advantage of them? How promptly or effectively have the community's members/hierarchy responded in providing consultation or emotional support to deal with the current health problem?

H. Has a counselor or advisor of that religious denomination been invited to provide guidance and support if the patient so wishes? Or for the health care team's information?

I. Are there special constraints or requirements imposed by the patient's religion on how the dying should be treated or how specifically to handle the body of a deceased with respect?

The patient's religion may, of course, be a critical element in how he interacts with the health care system. For example, in the treatment of the dying patient, the Jewish belief in the infinite value of life plays a vital part. According to the Talmud, "one who is in a dying condition is regarded as a living person in all respects." The condition is compared to a flickering flame inasmuch as, if one touches it, that flame might be extinguished. The patient in such a state, according to Orthodox Jewish tradition, may not be washed, his pillow may not be touched, his eyes may not be closed, and he may not be moved. In short, nothing should be done that might hasten his death. All efforts needed to protect and nourish the "flickering flame" must be undertaken. This may become a problem for an elderly Orthodox Jew, who is obviously terminally ill and dying in an Intensive Care Unit. For that patient (and/or his family) to permit his (the patient's) being moved would be a violation of Jewish law.

Under the heading of education and intelligence, the following questions may be appropriate to raise:

A. Has the patient received any education beyond the elementary grades?

B. Does accepting the current medical problem and complying with or participating in medical recommendations coordinate with the patient's level of education and intelligence?

C. Does the patient's behavior or practice deviate from his intellectual development, understanding, or past education?

In terms of work history or profession, additional questions might include the following:

A. Has the patient's prior profession or occupation been "at odds" with "medicine?" Has the patient, or a close member of the family, been a malpractice attorney, a chiropractor, Christian Science practitioner, or naturopath?

B. Has the patient been a "success" in his or her job, profession, or other activities, so that he or she has established some sense of self-esteem or self-worth? What constitutes or contributes to "self-worth" in that culture?

C. Does he or she, even subconsciously, feel that the disease or current clinical problem is a welcome relief and/or an excuse for past failures? May the disease be recognized as a justification for or explanation of them?

D. Is there an occupational relationship to the patient's disease? In other words, has this been a job-related injury or illness, and if so what is the patient's emotional response to it? Is he or she aware of this association? If not, should that information be communicated?

With respect to the patient's past encounters with the health care system, the team members should consider:

A. Has the patient been in the hospital before or previously been treated by this physician or team of health care providers?

B. Have prior experiences with the health care system been pleasant, effective, and marked with positive outcomes?

C. Was there relief of suffering provided in previous encounters along with a caring attitude, even though no cure was effected or possible?

D. Have prior encounters been distinguished by dissatisfaction, poor outcomes, a perception that the physician or other providers "didn't care," or were just interested in increasing the size of the patient's bill?

Similar questions might be posed with respect to prior encounters between the health care system and the patient's parents, spouse, children, other family members or friends. Certainly, if the patient or a family member has previously been involved in a malpractice suit, subsequent relationships with care providers might well be uncomfortable and adversely affect the provider-patient relationship. In such a situation, there may be a need to mediate lest potential hostility between the parties adversely affect the healing or support relationship.

In the context of lifestyle, the health care team member might inquire into the patient's hobbies, outside activities, tendencies toward a "workaholic" personality, or other incentives to "return" to a more active social life and prior relationships. The patient's past history as an active individual — sports, physical activities, health-promoting or healthful (as opposed to risk-taking) behaviors — is also important.

In terms of family relationships, it would be appropriate to ask about the closeness of the family, mutual respect, compatibility of interests and endeavors, conformity with past family beliefs and future family plans, particularly in terms of determining who should serve as an appropriate surrogate should the patient become incapable of participating personally in health care decisions. In this setting, clandestine relationships in which the patient may have been involved and about which the family may have no knowledge, i.e., homosexual, bi-sexual, or other socially stigmatized activities, may be critical in the decision-making process or in the search for an appropriate surrogate.

It is also important to inquire about the nature of the patient's own (as opposed to a cultural) perception of "illness" in contrast with "disease."

A. What meaning does the patient's overall illness/disease have at this point in his or her life?

B. What are the present symptoms, and what meaning do they have at this particular time?

C. How can the health care system best help him or her deal with them and resume his or her life/lifestyle in the most meaningful way, if that is possible?

In terms of the patient's sex, particularly if the patient is a female, cultural concerns and the relative role of females in that culture are critical. Among certain cultures, married females have no right to make decisions for themselves but must defer to their husbands. Similarly, adult unmarried women must defer to their parents or older brothers for decisions regarding their care and treatment. The "competent female adult" from that culture might never be asked her wishes; only male members of her family or her husband may describe her symptoms or consent to her treatment, depending on how closely she identifies with the culture of origin.

Varying perceptions regarding bodily integrity may also be of concern. For example, some cultures, particularly the Chinese, believe that the body is preserved in the "next life" essentially in the state in which it was buried. For patients from that culture to consent to elective or even emergency amputation or organ transplant, perceiving that they will survive in the hereafter without the amputated or removed body part or with someone else's organ might prove extremely distressful to them.

II. Critical Factors Concerning the Physician or Other Principal Health Care Provider

The cultural background of the physician or other closely involved care provider is also important in the communication with the patient. The physician's (or other provider's) own background and culture must not become so dominant that the patient and/or the family are afforded no opportunity to ask questions or obtain further information. Now that there are so many "minority cultures" in the United States, it is particularly important that the religious, cultural, national, or ethnic background of any of the providers not be permitted to disenfranchise the patient or the family (surrogates) and/or subvert their wishes. This is especially true if the patient has considered himself or herself in a subservient social class, perhaps less deserving and therefore more willing to suppress his or her own will or wishes (or those of the family), in deference to the physician or other health care provider who was perceived as being coercive, perhaps even unintentionally.

For example, the Orthodox Jewish physician may experience conflict from a religious standpoint in dealing with a patient on an emergency basis on the

Sabbath (e.g., responding to telephone calls, coming to the hospital to treat an emergency) or in treating a non-Jewish dying patient while acceding to the Orthodox Jewish belief in the infinite value of human life and the necessity to prolong life indefinitely.

In this context, the Orthodox Jewish definition of death may be critical. Judaism's criteria for death require the absence of spontaneous respiration and heartbeat in a patient with no bodily movement. Whether or not brain criteria for declaring death — defined as the totally irreversible cessation of all brain function, including the brain stem — should be applied may create a problem for the Orthodox physician in pronouncing a patient dead. This is especially true where the brain-dead patient still retains even minimal spinal reflexes. Also of importance here is the issue of the physician under such personal religious constraints seeking to apply "all heroic measures" to prolong life, especially in the case of a patient, not of the same religious persuasion, who might wish to refuse such treatment.

In that context, team members should assure themselves that the most intimately involved parties are aware of one another's points of view and are comfortable collaborating in that environment with those constraints. In some cases, a patient who represents an ethnic or religious minority and his or her physician may already have satisfactorily worked out the details of how treatment is to proceed. Team members may ascertain the facts and accordingly resist the temptation to question whether the patient's wishes are being respected and other ethical issues being addressed. Involvement by third parties in such cases may constitute an inappropriate and unwelcome intrusion into the provider-patient relationship, when no need or problem exists. Unfortunately, if this is not carefully worked out beforehand, the patient's confidence in the relationship with his physician may be disturbed. For instance, in certain Arabic and Semitic cultures, the physician is treated with the utmost respect and trust. For a physician to ask the patient or the family for a decision regarding the patient's future care would raise in their minds the thought that the physician was not competent or confident of the diagnosis or treatment plan. It would destroy the family's confidence in the physician and might totally disrupt the therapeutic relationship. Individuals from those cultures are usually very comfortable working with a physician who totally directs the course of treatment and finds no need for an information-giving dialogue or a consent-obtaining procedure. Patients do have the right to refuse to assert their autonomy and to follow the physician's suggestions without question.

With respect to the concept of "truth telling," there are certain ethnic, religious, and cultural groups among whom the diagnosis of cancer is never given or spoken, because it is presumed to telegraph a fatal and hopeless prognosis. Accordingly, the various members of the health care team may wish to assure that the patient's perception of the propriety and adequacy of communication of "acceptable" diagnoses, information, and consent is being met in an ongoing therapeutic relationship with caregivers. (This is especially the case among Russian and Japanese immigrants.)

III. The Nature of the Community

Similar questions might also be raised about the hospital itself, especially if it is owned by or affiliated with a particular religious, social, or community organization and therefore has its own pre-existing "agenda." Mechanisms should be established and implemented to assure that patients and their families are informed of institutional policies or positions on certain issues, e.g., therapeutic modalities provided, patients' rights, patients' relationship to the caregiver and/or the institution, etc.

The nature of the local community (whether it represents the culture, ethnicity, or religion of the patient and the family, or is significantly different) may also be a matter of concern. Health care team members themselves may have values which differ from the patient's and therefore find it difficult to comprehend his or her culture, wishes, past practices, and health care concerns. Hence, they must be especially cautious lest they be influenced unduly by their own particular backgrounds. They cannot be permitted to prejudice discussions with the patient or the care-giving process, nor to infringe upon the patient's rights or opportunity to have his or her own needs and wishes acknowledged. In other words, team members must conduct themselves and their professional activities ethically.

IV. Educational Efforts and Policy and Guideline Development

Opportunities should be provided for the entire health care staff to become familiar with the variety of cultures represented in the hospital's community and among its patient mix. Practitioners, spokespersons for the particular culture, or sociologists from local colleges or universities should be invited to meet with the administration, the Executive Board, the Medical and Nursing Staffs, and other members of the health care team to discuss issues of particular concern in the relevant ethnic settings. It is critical that staff members become comfortable with and work to understand the individual practices or beliefs of these groups.

From time to time, as particular situations arise, consultants might be invited to assist in policy development, to reinforce familiarity with the practices of the cultures or ethnic groups represented among the facility's patient mix, to make sure that patients of different cultures are treated in a setting and in a manner which makes them feel comfortable, i.e., in an environment where their wishes and needs are truly met. The educational process should be on-going. Lectures, small discussion groups, and reference materials in the library should be utilized to broaden the awareness of all involved.

Perhaps the most appropriate recommendation to make to team members is that they facilitate the preparation of a "Values History" or similar document for patients admitted to their facility. This may help assure that the patients' cultural backgrounds, beliefs, values and other aspects of their personhood are considered in providing their medical care and in reaching appropriate decisions regarding that care. The "Values History" can serve as a significant core of information about the patient and his or her particular orientation to help guide caregivers. A sample of such a "Values Document" follows. It has been adapted with permission from an instrument originally developed by Joan McIver Gibson, Ph.D., of the School of Law at the University of New Mexico in Albuquerque.

Summary

In the past, the United States has been characterized as a vast melting pot where the individual's culture of origin received little or no attention in the process of health care.

Recently, with the arrival of more and more diverse groups on our shores, there has been a great interest in fostering multicultural activities, with emphasis on a heightened awareness of our ethnic variety. At times of illness or accident, our vulnerability as individuals increases and our comfort is enhanced by the familiar, by the practices and behaviors with which we grew up and identify.

It therefore behooves those involved in health care to familiarize themselves with the cultures with which they come into contact in their professional activities, to maintain an open and inquiring mind, and to be willing to compromise to accommodate to the patient's needs, where possible. By enhancing and encouraging communication in this very vital area, the long-acknowledged goals of medicine and health care will be more readily achieved:

> to cure sometimes;
>
> to relieve often;
>
> to comfort always.

Suggested Outline for a "Values History" or "Values Document"

Written Wishes or Directives

1. Have wishes been expressed in terms of a Living Will, Directive to Physicians, Durable Power of Attorney, or other comparable legal documents?

2. Has the patient written anything regarding wishes about organ donation, dialysis, CPR, palliation, chemotherapy, radiation therapy, surgery, respirators, transfusions, artificial nutrition or hydration, or other "high tech" treatment modalities?

Oral Statements

1. Has the patient ever expressed him/herself *orally* to anyone, regarding any of the above?
2. In conversations with others about the patient's own attitudes toward health care, in what ways have existing medical problems appeared to restrict the patient's ability to function? What has been the patient's response to these restrictions?

Patient's Attitude Toward Personal Health and Health Care

1. How does the patient feel about his or her health? What is the patient's perception of the physician's role and responsibility in decision making or in information giving? What role or responsibility has the patient assumed in decisions regarding health in the past? Has it changed with the present illness or clinical problem? Has the patient formally deferred to others in the past to make these decisions? To what extent are persistent or intractable pain, disability or dependence factors in the current clinical situation?
2. What has been the nature of the patient's previous encounter(s) with the health care system, and with physicians in particular? Favorable? Poor? How well did he or she adapt to the illness? Or to its "bad outcomes?" What has been the nature of previous encounters with the health care system by the patient's family members? Friends? Did the patient or family initiate any malpractice litigation?

Patient's Attitude Toward His or Her Life

1. What is the extent of the patient's education? Intelligence? What activities, relationships, and hobbies have been important to the patient? How does the patient feel about what he or she has accomplished in life — career, contributions, other "successes," participation in family, group, or community achievements? What are present aspirations and goals? Do personal goals remain unfulfilled? Are these realistically attainable, in whole or in part?
2. What are the patient's fears? How important has it been both in the past and at present for the patient to maintain independence and control over

his or her life? Who or what have been the dominant persons/elements in the patient's life? Are current frustrations or disappointments factors?

3. How can one best describe the patient's relationships with his family? With friends? Caregivers? The attending physician? What important personal or interpersonal issues is the patient coping with at this time?

Religion and Personal Philosophy

1. What are the patient's basic beliefs about God or a transcendent power? What are the patient's ties (past and present) with particular churches, denominations, healers, priests, ministers or rabbis? What is the role of prayer, sacrament, sacrifice, "penance," "guilt" in the patient's life? What meaning, if any does the patient ascribe to death? To an afterlife?

2. What feelings does the patient have about illness, suffering, and dying generally? What meaning does the patient ascribe to his or her illness? What does the patient fear most about the illness or condition? How does he or she view *his or her dying*? What wishes has the patient made known regarding arrangements after death—funeral, cremation, memorial services? Has he or she prepared a will or otherwise disposed of possessions?

3. If the patient has been told that death is imminent, what is the response? How would one best describe the patient's current mind-set? Denial/depression/anger/bargaining/acceptance?

Bibliography

Anderson, J. N. 1983. "Health and Illness in Philippino Immigrants." *Western Journal of Medicine,* 139:811-19.

Banatar, S. R. 1988. "Ethics, Medicine, and Health in South Africa." *Hastings Center Report* 4, Supplement, 18:3-8.

Berlin, E. A., and Fowkes, W. C. 1983. "A Teaching Framework for Cross-Cultural Health Care — Application and Family Practice." *Western Journal of Medicine,* 139:934-38.

Book, P. A., Dixon, M., and Karchner, S. 1983. "Native Healing in Alaska — Report from Serpentine Hotsprings." *Western Journal of Medicine,* 139:923-27.

Brodsky, C. M. 1983. "Culture and Disability Behavior." *Western Journal of Medicine,* 139:892-99.

Clark, M. 1983. "Cultural Context of Medical Practice." *Western Journal of Medicine,* 139:806-10.

Clark, M. 1970. "Health in the Mexican-American Culture." University of California Press, Berkeley.

Dracopoulou, S., and Doxiadis, S. 1988. "Care of the Dying — In Greece, Lament for the Dead, Denial for the Dying." *Hastings Center Report,* 4, Supplement, 18:15-16.

Fitzpatrick-Nietschmann, J. 1983. "Pacific Islanders — Migration and Health." *Western Journal of Medicine*, 139:848-53.

Franca, O. 1988. "In Uruguay, An Ethic of Care for the Dying." *Hastings Center Report*, 4, Supplement, 18:21-22.

Freimer, N., Echenberg, D., and Kretchmer, N. 1983. "Cultural Variation — Nutritional and Clinical Applications." *Western Journal of Medicine*, 139:928-33.

Gonzalez-Lee, T. and Simon, H. J. 1987. "Teaching Spanish and Cross-Cultural Sensitivity to Medical Students." *Western Journal of Medicine*, 146:502-4.

Hartog, J. and Hartog, E. A. 1983. "Cultural Aspects of Health and Illness Behavior in Hospitals." *Western Journal of Medicine*, 139:910-12.

Hermeren, G. 1988. "In Sweden, Questioning the Model of Compromise." *Hastings Center Report*, 4, Supplement, 18:17-18.

Kim, S. S. 1983. "Ethnic Elders and American Health Care — A Physican's Perspective." *Western Journal of Medicine*, 139:885-91.

Kleinman, A. 1980. "Patients and Healers in the Context of Culture." University of California Press, Berkeley.

Lefevre, C. 1988. "In France, Terminal Stage Medicine is not Hopelessly Ill." *Hastings Center Report*, 4, Supplement, 18:19-20.

Lin, T. Y. 1983. "Psychiatry and Chinese Culture." *Western Journal of Medicine*, 139:862-67.

Lipson, J. G., and Meleis, A. I. 1983. "Issues and Health Care of Middle Eastern Patients." *Western Journal of Medicine*, 139:854-61.

Llano-Escobar, A. 1988. "In Columbia, Dealing with Death and Technology." *Hastings Center Report*, 4, Supplement, 18:23-24.

Maduro, R. 1983. "Curanderismo and Latino Views of Disease and Curing." *Western Journal of Medicine*, 139:868-74.

Meleis, A. I. 1979. "The Health Care System of Kuwait: The Social Paradoxes." *Social Science and Medicine*, 13A:743-49.

Meleis, A. I. and Jonsen, A. R. 1983. "Ethical Crises and Cultural Differences." *Western Journal of Medicine*, 138:889-91.

Mitchell, M. F. 1983. "Popular Medical Concepts in Jamaica and Their Impact on Drug Use." *Western Journal of Medicine*, 139:841-47.

Muecke, M. A. 1983. "In Search of Healers — Southeast Asian Refugees and the American Health Care System." *Western Journal of Medicine*, 139:835-40.

Racy, J. 1969. "Death in an Arab Culture." *Annals New York Academy of Sciences*, 164:871-80.

"Religious Aspects of Medical Care — A Handbook of Religious Practices of All Faiths, 2nd Ed." 1978. The Catholic Hospital Association, St. Louis, MO.

Saunders, L. 1954. "Cultural Difference in Medical Care." Russell Sage Foundation, New York.

Snow, L. F. 1983. "Traditional Health Beliefs in Practices Among Lower Class Black Americans." *Western Journal of Medicine*, 139:820-28.

Tranoy, K. E. 1988. "Bio-medical Value Conflict." *Hastings Center Report*, 4, Supplement, 18:8-10.

The Value of Many Voices. 1987. Summary of a Conference on Cultural, Religious, Social and Economic Differences that Complicate Health Care; Abrams, F. R. and

Reiquam, C. W., Co-facilitators, Center for Health Ethics and Policy, University of Colorado at Denver Graduate School of Public Affairs, Denver, CO.

Veatch, R. M. 1989. "Medical Ethics in the Soviet Union." *Hastings Center Report,* 2, 19:11-14.

Wolf, S. M., and Donnelley, S. 1988. "Doing Ethics in Italy." *Hastings Center Report,* 4, Supplement, 18:13-14.

Ethical Communication in Health Care

Ethics govern the moral acceptability of behavior in different social contexts. Ethical positions such as standards for health behaviors, are established through interaction within a given community and are often culturally-bound. For example, there are religious, legal (national and regional), and professional standards, codes, oaths, and principles for the ways in which health care providers and consumers are to interact with one another. Ethical standards in health care govern such issues as confidentiality, informed consent, health care decision making, the preservation of life, and the rights of different, often disenfranchised, populations of consumers (such as the elderly, the disabled, the dying, women, and children).

Unfortunately, ethical standards are not always communicated very clearly within different communities and these standards can be easily and unintentionally violated. Moreover, when people from different cultural orientations

179

interact, as they often do in health care, moral dilemmas arise where there are contradictory cultural values guiding the health care decisions in which providers and consumers engage.

Communication about ethical issues enables health care providers and consumers to recognize and evaluate ethical constraints on their behaviors. Through interaction these health care participants can adjust their behaviors to meet each other's expectations and establish common ground for overcoming moral dilemmas. Kreps and Thornton (1992) suggest a plan called the ESSAA method (ESSAA stands for ethical readiness, sorting, solving, acting, and assessing) for promoting ethical action. This section of the book examines several ethical communication issues in modern health care and suggests strategies for promoting ethical behavior in health care.

The first reading in this chapter entitled "Blowing the Whistle" is an article written by Barbara Thornton that was originally published in *California Nursing Review*. In the reading, Thornton discusses the many communication problems that arise when it is not possible to utilize conventional organizational channels to solve moral dilemmas. The reading begins with an account of a brutal case of professional misconduct and sexual assault and then describes the difficulties of reporting such abuses. The reading describes how and when to "blow the whistle" on unethical behavior in health care, as well as how to cover yourself and gather needed social support.

The second reading, written by Barbara Thornton, Rosalie Marinelli, and Trudy Larson, examines many of the ethical concerns women face in the modern health care system. This article clearly illustrates the ethical issues that arise when different cultures (in this case male culture and female culture) conflict. This reading identifies the many disturbing inequities women face within the health care system and concludes by suggesting strategies for empowering female health care consumers to take charge of their own health care and resist being abused by the health care system.

The third reading, "Communicating About Death" written by Gary Kreps, examines the difficulties Americans experience in confronting and discussing death. Kreps identifies several culturally-based reasons for these difficulties and describes many of the ways we avoid frank and honest communication about death and dying. The reading concludes by suggesting strategies for communicating therapeutically to help people demystify death and overcome their fears. How comfortable are you taking about death? Are there certain people with whom you feel comfortable talking about death and others who make you feel uncomfortable? Why?

Kreps, G. L. & Thornton, B. C. (1992). *Health Communication: Theory and Practice* 2nd edition. Prospect Heights, IL: Waveland Press.

17

Blowing the Whistle

By Barbara C. Thornton

You are a surgical nurse who has just seen an anesthesiologist sexually assault an unconscious patient. You suspect the administration as well as your superiors will not listen to your report, as he is both prominent and powerful in the medical community. What do you do?

This case actually occurred in California some years ago, and it reflects the lonely and difficult dilemma faced by nurses as well as other professionals as they confront a process known as "*whistle-blowing.*" While the term is sometimes found offensive, no other terminology has been utilized to describe the circumstance in which an individual finds it necessary to share information about a situation or a person outside the normal reporting channels. "Whistle-blower" is the label attached to those who call attention to negligence, abuses, or dangers which threaten the public. Whistle-blowing is accomplished by going outside the system to report wrongdoing, and such a process usually occurs when the internal organization is seen as an ineffective or dangerous place in which to share information.

Whistle-blowing is particularly difficult because it involves an ethical conflict of duties. The professional feels responsible to patients as well as to colleagues, and when these responsibilities appear to be in conflict, an ethical tension develops. This tension is not resolved by most codes of ethics which stress accountability to the public but do not establish the principles and procedures to be utilized when it is necessary to expose wrongdoing.

Writers on the health professions, such as Eliot Friedson (1961), maintain that the values of the health care professional as reflected in codes often do not advocate for the patient's best interests but express the loyalty of the individual to the profession and to each other. A breach of loyalty which implies dissent or accusation is particularly threatening to one's core group.

A version of this article appeared in the *California Nursing Review,* 10 (1988): 24-27. The article elicited the most "Letters to the Editor" in the journal's history. For assistance regarding whistle-blowing procedures, contact Don Soeken, Integrity International, 6215 Greenbelt Road, Suite 102, College Park, MD 20740; (301) 953-7358.

In addition to raising the issue of conflict of duties, whistle-blowing also involves ethical virtues such as courage. Certainly, in recent times, a whistle-blower who is acting out of altruism is often thought of as courageous, and many proponents see such action as benevolent or caring. Other principles which are the basis for exposing wrongdoing are: concern for patient autonomy; animosity toward paternalistic action; and, truthtelling. A sense of justice is also an ethical consideration.

Well-Known Whistle-Blowers

Whistle-blowing became more prominent in the 1960s in many of the professions and in business. Seen as an outgrowth of the consumer protection and civil rights movements, some employees began to argue for more accountability. Karen Silkwood, who accused the Kerr-McGee chemical plant of mishandling plutonium; Ernest Fitzgerald, who blew the whistle on Pentagon overruns; and Frank Serpico, who exposed corruption in the New York Police Department, are examples of well-known whistle-blowers who exemplified courage and an ethical concern for the public (McGowan, 1984; Westin, 1981).

In health care, nurses and other health professionals have triggered investigations in such areas as euthanasia, the care of neonates (particularly those born with disabling conditions) and sexual misconduct. One of the most prominent of the latter cases, the Miofsky case, which was referred to at the beginning of this article, took place in California in the late 1970s. Investigations resulted in national criticism of the medical profession, once it was discovered that healthcare professionals had prior knowledge of Dr. Miofsky's sexual conduct and had not immediately reported it (Clark & Shapiro, 1979).

When and How to Blow the Whistle

What are the consequences for a health professional who is seriously troubled by the wrongdoing that he or she has observed on the part of others? What happens when action is taken which might result in the loss of a job as well as intense criticism by colleagues or the denouncement by one's superiors? Newspapers are full of stories which tell about retaliation taken against those who share information outside normal channels.

One of the purposes of this article is to briefly outline the suggestions for a procedure that would be helpful to someone contemplating the need to report a potential wrongdoing. While this task is never easy, the following guidelines have been used by others or suggested by experts in this field. Certainly they will need to be tailored to fit the particular case.

Before proceeding to share the information you have, you need to determine the ethical reason for contemplating your action. According to Sissela Bok, in her fine book *Secrets* (1982), it is clearly inappropriate to expose legitimate private matters which have to do with political beliefs or one's personal sexual life. Ask yourself if you are sincerely acting on behalf of patients and their families rather than a concern for your own interests. If the answer is yes, you have a strong reason for proceeding.

Once the facts are checked out and you are confident you can handle the conflicts and possible harassment which might arise, you need to investigate your institution's procedures. Organizations have historically been reluctant to provide protection to the whistle-blower, but this is changing. If possible, you need to air your complaint to someone who can listen carefully, who has the power to check out the situation and do something about it, and who can protect and support you. If this person does not exist within the organization, is he or she available in another setting?

It is at this point that several other kinds of people need to be identified who could also assist you. Is there another health professional who might be willing to help you collect the facts? It is much more difficult for the administration to ignore a group of health professionals than just one person. It is particularly powerful for you to have the corroboration of others if you are bringing charges against a physician or administrator who has more power in the organization than you do. Other people, if they are willing, can also help you explore alternative ways within the organization to handle the problem with diplomacy, creativity, and brainstorming, since whistle-blowing should be a last resort. Don Soeken recommends being as detached and as realistic as possible (McGowan, 1984).

Support Systems

Whether acting alone or in concert, whistle-blowers need to have a personal support system. Even though the reputation of whistle-blowers is changing in a positive direction, still there are situations in which they are called trouble-makers. It is important to have support in maintaining your psychological stability, especially if retaliation takes place. Psychiatric social worker Don Soeken says that the whistle-blower needs assistance with stress reduction. Seeking the advice of a good counselor is helpful. This person can help review the event with you as well as the ethical and psychological reasons for the whistle-blowing. He or she can also support you as you understand and deal with the immense power that can be used against a person bucking the system. It is also advisable to work with someone who understands the legal consequences and can help you get publicity, if that is necessary.

Sharing the Information

Once your support system is in place, you will want to begin the process of sharing your information with the appropriate sources. If possible, select several people you can contact. It is sometimes helpful if they are in different settings. Not only will this allow you to get diverse reactions, it will also give you additional support. Present your facts as carefully as possible and stay as personally detached as you can manage. Stress the adverse effects you feel that the wrongdoing will have on patients and colleagues. Present a suggested plan of action if you have one and agree with your contact on how you will proceed.

Leaking the information to the news media is a possibility many people consider — particularly because it is less dangerous to the informer. *Deep Throat*, for example, the whistle-blower who leaked information during the Watergate scandal has never been absolutely identified. There are problems with leaking material, however, because once leaked, the information is out of control and can be utilized haphazardly and even irresponsibly.

After all your efforts to collect evidence, ask questions, and select contacts, your attempts to correct the wrongdoing still might not be successful. Your complaint can die in the hands of the people you thought would help you. You can be fired in states which do not have adequate legislation to protect you, or you can be demoted or reassigned to an unsuitable position. That's why it is important to prepare for adverse consequences by developing alternative job plans.

With such potential for adversity, why would anyone undertake such action? The answer is straightforward for someone who sees a wrong being committed and a patient being harmed. Living with the guilt of not doing the right thing leads to a sense of self-condemnation or moral pain which is often more difficult than the consequences of the whistle-blowing.

Developing Responsible Systems

Because the life of the whistle-blower is not an easy one and because a democratic society should not encourage the hiding of information harmful to patients or consumers, professional groups need to develop procedures before incidents of wrongdoing occur. For example, an organization can reduce the need to blow the whistle by having open channels for evaluating criticism. Those who are seen as having less power than physicians and administrators in the health care system should be particularly motivated to work for state legislation and institutional safeguards that will protect their members as they carry out their patient advocacy tasks. Strong and clear procedures which protect the whistle-blower need to be established which encourage accountability and deter wrongdoing. It goes without saying that these same statutes should protect the accused unless they are proven guilty.

Suggestions for Specific Changes

First and foremost, confidentiality has to be assured to persons who file a report. Such confidentiality keeps names out of the investigative process and avoids personal animosity and interpersonal conflict while the facts are being investigated. Procedures can be established whereby the person making the report can be protected until a preliminary investigation has been completed. If it is then determined that the charges have a basis for further examination, the person accused should have access to information which might include appropriate accessibility to the person making the accusation. Some whistle-blowing advocates argue, however, that the whistle-blower's confidentiality should always be protected if whistle-blowing is to become a sanctioned and useful mechanism for the safety and well-being of society.

Most importantly, health professionals need to work for legislation such as the Michigan Whistle-blowing Protection Act which makes it illegal for a Michigan employer to retaliate against a worker who reports or is about to report a suspected violation of federal, state or local law. This law, which has already made it easier for persons to pursue wrongdoing, indicates that whistle-blowing is finally recognized as an activity which provides benefits to society.

Society's Values

Finally, we have to look at the general values held by society. At a conference on whistle-blowing one of the participants noted that we educate our children to be good little politicians who are inculcated to play along at very early ages. "Tell the truth, but don't — for God's sake — tell it out loud in the wrong place at the wrong time!" We, in effect, discourage whistle-blowing from a very early age. With these conditions, the participant noted, we shouldn't be surprised if whistle-blowers are regarded as poor sports. However, moral life is not made for our convenience, and society needs to train its young to be truthful as well as to support people of courage who dare to make a difference.

References

Bok, S. (1982). *Secrets: On the ethics of concealment and revelation.* New York: Random House.

Clark, M. and Shapiro, D. (1979, April 16). Disciplining doctors. *Newsweek,* 93:66.

Friedson, E.(1961). *Patients' views of medical practice.* N.Y.: Sage Foundation.

McGowan, W. (1984, November 25). Whistle-blowing: Truth or Consequences. This World Supplement. *San Francisco Chronicle,* 9-12.

Westin, A. F. (1981). *Whistle-blowing: Loyalty and dissent in the corporation.* N.Y.: McGraw-Hill.

18

Ethics and Women's Health Care
By *Barbara C. Thornton, Rosalie D. Marinelli* and *Trudy Larson*

Women's Health Care

Health care as well as health-care ethics (more commonly known as bioethics) are fields that have been dominated by men. One of the positions of this article is that women and men do not make ethical decisions in the same manner. Therefore, a system dominated by male decision makers is not providing a female view of health care.

If women are viewed as "other" (that is, different from men), the male model becomes the standard, and women are seen in relation to that standard. According to this view, women become deviant or different from the norm when they are involved in reproductive functions. If reproduction, on the other hand, was seen as a unique and important phenomenon rather than a deviation from maleness, women and their reproductive health would be treated differently (Eisenstein, 1988).

The model by which we view women and their health, influences both the patient and the health-care provider in their ethical and diagnostic decision making. It has long been argued that women are at a disadvantage in health care because they are not a major part of health care decision making. While women were 60 percent of the patient population and 80 percent of the nursing home patients, they were, in 1988, only 15 percent of active physicians, the group that still makes most of the health-care decisions (Friedman, 1988, p. 681). Although this number is steadily growing, noticeable differences in women's empowerment as patients or physicians have not, as yet, occurred.

A tightening of Medicaid qualifications has resulted in the loss of coverage for many poor women and their children. Medicaid, at one time, provided coverage for 65 percent of the poor in the United States. But recent figures

A version of this article appeared in *Choices and Challenges: The Nevada Public Affairs Review* (1990, pp. 20-24). The authors are members of the faculty at the University of Nevada, Reno.

estimate that only 38 percent are covered. These limitations on care particularly affect minority women and single women who are heads of families (Braveman, et al., 1988).

The Political Context

National and world political views have also been major factors influencing women. Hans Morgenthau (1978), a well known scholar of world politics, said that if a nation needs manpower (usually to fight wars) it will exert more control over its female population by establishing laws and customs that encourage reproduction and family life. If there is a population explosion, the nation encourages the opposite.

Contemporary examples of this include overpopulated China, which has a one-child-per-family policy because of the need that country has to reduce its population growth, and underpopulated Romania, which until recently used state resources to insure that women became pregnant as often as possible. These examples demonstrate how decisions, often thought of as belonging to the individual or family, are influenced by the larger political context.

Five major concerns raised by critics of the historical models of health care are:

1. Physicians do not take women's complaints seriously.
2. The male patient is used as the standard in research and practice.
3. Women are subjected to excessive surgical procedures.
4. Women are often prescribed excessive amounts of drugs by their physicians.
5. Sexism and sexist models still dominate medical schools and health-care institutions.

Whether these concerns will be seriously addressed as women gain more power in health care is still to be determined. In 1949 only 11 percent of the graduates of medical schools were women, compared to 37 percent in 1988. For every eight college women who want to be nurses, ten want to be physicians, and women now comprise 51 percent of first-year residents in obstetrics and gynecology. Females also comprise 80 percent of the health-care work force including nurses, although they are still not often found in powerful positions (Friedman, 1988).

As more women become physicians, studies indicate some important differences from males. While the technical skill of both genders is similar, women physicians seem better able to communicate sensitivity and caring to patients. They listen without interrupting, they allow patients to present their agendas, and they develop stronger rapport by providing more time for discussion. Additionally, they are more willing to have egalitarian relationships with patients. These studies also suggest that better physician-patient relationships lead to improved patient care (Arnold, Martin and Parker, 1988).

It is hoped that eventually the training of women and men physicians will support a caring, nurturing society and that there will be less conflict for women physicians in training where they will not be expected to become "one of the guys." Within this environment, it is hoped that patients' concerns will be listened to more closely, with greater credence, and will result in more patient-directed approaches. Patients, both male and female, will benefit greatly if these changes continue.

Ethical Concerns of Women

While ethics has received increased attention in recent years, specific women's ethical issues and their ethical decision making styles have been largely ignored. In the following sections of this article we will analyze some of these issues and talk about decision making. Our focus will be on the ethical principles of autonomy and paternalism, doing good (beneficence) and doing no harm (nonmaleficence) as well as justice and the allocation of resources.

Autonomy and Paternalism

The autonomy and paternalism debate concerns all patients. Autonomy indicates that persons of sound mind should be able to make decisions regarding their own bodies. This right has been upheld by the courts, based particularly on the doctrine of informed consent. The opposite of autonomy is paternalism, which is making decisions for someone incapable of making them for himself or herself. The issues of autonomy and paternalism are of particular concern in regard to women and reproduction.

Much of the debate surrounding reproductive rights has to do with the perception of many health care providers and policy makers that pregnancy is an aberration, somehow affecting the competency of women. This paternalistic opinion is unconvincing as pregnancy is a natural state through which women are very functional.

Recent cases of forced caesarean sections are particularly illustrative. Angela Carter, a 28-year-old woman with cancer became pregnant; she stopped chemotherapy for the sake of the baby and decided to continue the pregnancy as normally as possible, hoping to deliver a viable infant. Her situation became precarious and a Caesarean section was recommended. The mother refused the surgery because she thought it was too soon to deliver the baby. Her family agreed, but a court order was issued by a judge who felt the benefit to the fetus superseded the mother's refusal. The Caesarean was performed and both the mother and the very premature infant died (Annas, 1988).

In analyzing this case, it is difficult to comprehend why the competent mother was given no consideration in the final decision. The judge authorizing the surgery did not consult her. "Treating the fetus against the will of the mother degrades and dehumanizes the mother and treats her as an inert container" (Annas, 1988, p. 24). On appeal, long after the mother and baby died, the District of Columbia Court of Appeals reversed this decision and reinforced the idea that competent patients should make decisions about all procedures and interventions, whether they are pregnant or not.

The related issue in this case is the right of a mature, competent woman to refuse surgery because of what she determined as the best interest of the fetus versus the decisions of health providers who had differing views. The viability of a fetus is unpredictable with current knowledge. Infants born very prematurely can be saved in some cases but with prolonged, and often painful, hospitalization. Certainly the decision, in such difficult circumstances, belongs with the woman, if informed consent applies equally to both genders.

Another well publicized case involved Nancy Klein, a pregnant woman who was in a coma as a result of an automobile accident. Her physicians felt the pregnancy might be hindering her recovery and recommended termination of the pregnancy to optimize her medical condition. Her husband agreed, and signed the permit. A pro-life activist group sought legal guardianship of Nancy Klein and her unborn child to prevent the abortion. The court in this instance ruled in favor of the husband, an abortion was performed, and the woman is slowly recovering (*New York Times*, February 12, 1989).

Issues involving surrogacy and in vitro fertilization are also of increasing concern for many women. Policy makers are seeking to determine the "rightful" parent in cases where women carry fetuses to term for other families. Many feminists disagree with the view that allows "a womb for rent" mentality which reduces pregnancy to a manufacturing analogy where the womb is the "container" and the baby the "product." It is particularly disturbing to many women that male judges who have not gone through pregnancy or childbirth establish laws in these areas.

The issues surrounding maternal and fetal health care are complex and reflect a struggle in reconciling technological medical advances with the basic human rights of people. The examples illustrate the precariousness of the rights of women, particularly pregnant women, in the struggle between paternalism and autonomy.

Doing Good and Doing No Harm

Doing good (beneficence) and doing no harm (nonmaleficence) have always played an important part in medical care and these principles are stressed in codes of ethics of the various health care disciplines. The difficulty of putting them into practice becomes glaringly evident in some of the issues facing women.

Two major issues serve to illustrate this. The abuse or battery of women and children has been handled typically from a "do no harm" standpoint rather than in the more assertive "do good" stance. The burden of proof is on the victim to prove battery occurred. Authorities, including medical authorities, have often felt it best not to step into the personal lives of families. There has been great leniency in domestic violence cases. In several cases, women have registered multiple complaints with the police, citing death threats, and evidence of battery. The complaints were usually ignored or minimized by the police, who used the right of privacy to justify nonintervention. Several of these women were subsequently murdered.

In rape cases, the rights of victims are often ignored, and the attitude that women are deliberately provocative discourages victims from coming forward to press charges. Even when the victims are determined enough to press charges against their attackers, the treatment they receive in court is disturbing. In four recent cases in New York City, the Central Park jogger, the "preppie" murder, the model whose face was brutally slashed, as well as the Kennedy Estate rape case in Florida, the victims became the targets of racist and sexist accusations. The victims, again brutalized by defense lawyers, the press and the public, had to defend their reputations and their lifestyles.

Spouse abuse, usually a phenomenon of violence against women, remains largely unrecognized by medical institutions. Yet women who are victims of violence more often turn to their physicians for help rather than to psychiatrists, social agencies, police officers or lawyers. The medical community can be an important resource for women who are victims of violence if health care providers would use their influence to make an impact on this problem (Burge, 1989).

The epidemic of AIDS also illustrates the medical complexities of the "do good" versus "do no harm" issue. When a person tests positive for HIV (the human immunodeficiency virus which causes AIDS) the information is usually confidential, protected from discovery by others unless the tested person signs a release of information. However, since HIV is sexually transmitted, the partners of the HIV-infected person may be similarly infected or at risk of infection and be totally unaware of their risk.

The dilemma pits the right of confidentiality of the patient against public health, or specifically, the duty to warn a potential victim. Some women unknowingly have sexual partners who are bisexual or use intravenous drugs, both risks to the women. A physician must weigh the rights of the HIV patient to confidentiality (do good for that patient) against the risk to the sexual partner (do no harm). Many states are addressing this issue through public health laws allowing disclosure of information to unknowing partners since HIV infection has such dire consequences.

Justice and the Doctor-Patient Relationship

Justice, which is equitability in health care, is the basis of the American system of law and of ethics. It is important to remember that justice is often interpreted differently by judges in different sections of the country as well as by individuals. Consequently it is often difficult to translate justice into legislation that is agreeable to all. The issue of abortion is illustrative.

Since abortion raises the issue of individual rights, shadowed by religious and sometimes cultural tradition, this is a particularly difficult issue to resolve. Do fetal rights supersede maternal rights? If a woman is pregnant and of sound mind, does she have the right to decide what happens to her body particularly when her dilemma is whether to continue her pregnancy or abort?

Are there situations where a woman should have this decision taken out of her hands? The answer is divided and varies across the courts of the country although in areas of health care other than reproduction, competent patients' rights to make their own decisions have been upheld. Feminists and other groups strongly argue that the right of the woman to make these decisions is paramount, particularly in a society that does little to assist women or families in the raising of children once they are born. A more conservative position maintains that fetuses should also have rights. For this reason the issues of abortion and birth control are still highly controversial ones in our society.

Justice and its ramifications pervade the doctor-patient relationship. This relationship rests on a fundamental trust and is further formalized by a set of guidelines, defined in law, which seeks to further this trust. Informed consent, confidentiality, and patient rights are important. Women have often suffered from an unequal status in the doctor-patient relationship affecting fairness in many aspects of the relationship. Little girls are often given inadequate genital exams; teenagers are poorly educated about birth control and women throughout their lifespan are not well educated about their bodies. Often an unsatisfactory doctor-patient relationship results in women of any age not being able to disclose concerns about sexuality or abuse.

The same is true in discussion of issues facing females as they grow older. Brief or nonexistent discussions of premenstrual syndrome, menstruation and menopause by health care providers minimizes the importance of these issues. When more invasive procedures may be indicated, such as hysterectomy or mastectomy, there historically has been inadequate information for true informed consent to be obtained. Hysterectomy has classically been treated as an operation of minor significance by the medical establishment even though recent studies suggest tremendous psychological impact including loss of libido, sexual dysfunction, and depression (Boston Women's Health Collective, 1984). These side effects are not adequately addressed by most physicians who have been trained to minimize or ignore these issues. In France, approximately one-third the rate of hysterectomies are performed compared to the United States, yet morbidity and mortality rates are similar (Payer, 1988).

Recent data indicate that mastectomy, particularly radical mastectomy, is not indicated in many cases of breast cancer. Studies have shown that lumpectomy (removal of the lump) combined with radiation therapy may be as effective as the physically disfiguring radical procedure. These options may not be adequately presented to the patient by a physician who believes that mastectomy is more effective. This lack of information significantly affects informed consent and does not allow for a patient to exercise her rights, even though patients have the right to make decisions felt by others to be "wrong." Justice is definitely not served through an unequal, uninformed doctor-patient relationship (Brenner, 1988).

Issues of justice change throughout a woman's life span. Small girls must worry about child abuse. Teenagers need information on reproduction, particularly on contraception and sexuality. Middle-aged and older women, who often provide the major caretaking responsibilities for both the younger and older members of families, are often faced with ethical decisions for self and others. In a society that does not provide monetary or social assistance to those providing the burden of caring, justice is often unavailable.

Allocation of Resources

Allocation of resources is an issue also associated with justice because it refers to the way goods are dispensed in a society. In the 1960s, women began to realize that health care resources were unfairly distributed. The issue is current today as maternal-fetal, home health-care, teenage sexuality, and other programs primarily affecting women are nonexistent or underfunded. A recent review of health insurance figures indicated that women have less health insurance than men, and those with the greatest needs have less financial access to health care. Gaps between whites and minorities are widening (Braveman, Olivia, Grisham-Miller, Schaff and Reiter, December 1988).

Since the patients with the greatest need for services in the future will be elderly women with chronic conditions, additional resources will also have to be available for service and research needs. The ethical question arises as to whether justice will be done in finding and allocating such resources to meet women's needs in all phases of the life span. Male legislators, judges, health administrators and researchers have not given these issues high priority in the past.

A National Institute of Health advisory committee reported in 1987 that less than 13.5 percent of the institute's nearly $6 billion budget was spent on women's health although women make up over 50 percent of the population. Additionally, $77 million a year is spent researching ways to prevent breast cancer (which strikes 1 in 9 women), compared with $648 billion spent on heart disease research, which primarily effects males (Grande, 1990). These issues are compounded by the fact that most politicians, policy makers and researchers are males. While a federal office of Research on Women's Health has recently been established, it will be many years before the gap in research and research funding for women's health will be narrowed (Women: The road ahead, 1991).

Women as Unique Ethical Decision Makers

As we address the ethical issues that particularly affect women in our society, it is interesting to note that a body of literature is developing regarding the question of whether women make the same kinds of ethical decisions as men. The assumption, until recently, has been that they do.

Moral reasoning in recent years has been associated primarily with Lawrence Kohlberg, a Harvard professor, who studied moral development. Kohlberg described six stages of moral development. He saw enlightened ethical decision makers as persons who could rank values on a hierarchy and dispense justice fairly. However, Carol Gilligan, one of the researchers working with Kohlberg, began to find different interpretations of their similar research. Gilligan, interviewing groups of women, including a group that had abortions, realized there were gender differences.

The women in Gilligan's studies were much more concerned about the effect of the ethical decisions on their relationships than they were about a hierarchy of principles. They focused on how their decisions would influence others in their network of family and friends. Gilligan contends that such relationship thinking is as important as the dispensing of justice (Gilligan, 1982).

Nel Nodding (1982) added to Gilligan's work by stressing that caring should be taught, beginning at birth, and that educated caring should permeate all levels of society. Nodding argues that you cannot make unethical decisions if you really care about those involved. She suggests that men as well as women can be taught to care so that both can become caregivers as well as caretakers. Caring is not just another variable or theory, but can best be seen as a process which needs to be learned and applied in health care and all other areas of life.

Empowering People Regarding Their Own Health Care

Empowering people to make wise, ethical decisions regarding health care involves insuring that they are assertive and knowledgeable. All patients need to understand their rights as well as their responsibilities in the health-care system. Local libraries (including medical libraries at hospitals or medical schools) contain a great deal of information on ethical decision making. A book on patient decision making by Tom and Celia Scully (1989), is particularly helpful.

Additionally, in order to make sound ethical decisions, patients need to establish such habits as taking well-thought-out lists of questions to the doctor's office. For example, a woman facing a hysterectomy or a caesarean needs to ask how many of these operations are done in the regions in which she lives, whether or not the physician feels a bias toward one procedure or another, and how much the physician believes in patient autonomy or shared decision making.

Another resource for the patient, female or male, is the patient advocate. Some health-care institutions provide such a service and some families or friends have learned to be advocates for each other, asking the hard questions and writing down the answers while the patient deals directly with the physician. Learning about available health education programs and studying the different technical and ethical views of various health-care providers are all an important part of being an educated, ethical consumer of health care.

Family members need to make their desires about their health care known to others through advanced directives such as living wills and durable powers of attorney, documents that assert their wishes and empower someone to carry out these wishes if they are ever incapacitated. Additionally, they need to know about ethics committees, located in most major hospitals, which will assist individuals and families in making health-care decisions, particularly those regarding death and termination of treatment.

Women also need to be more assertive socially and politically. The most current successful political model was developed by the advocates of more funding for HIV research and the care and treatment of persons with AIDS. Women (and those who care about them) need to utilize the same techniques by impressing policy makers with the importance of their vital health care concerns. Health care ethicists also have an obligation to make women's health care issues a major agenda item.

Bibliography

Annas, G. 1988. She's going to die: The case of Angela C. *The Hastings Center Report*, 18, 23-25.

Arnold, R. M., Martin, S. C. and Parker, R. 1988. Taking care of patients—Does it matter whether the physician is a woman? *The Western Journal of Medicine*, 149:729-733.

The Boston Women's Health Collective. 1984. *The New Our Bodies, Ourselves*. New York: Simon and Schuster.

Braveman, P., Olivia, G., Grisham-Miller, M., Schaff, V. M. and Reiter, R. 1988. Women without health insurance: Links between access, poverty, ethnicity and health. *The Western Journal of Medicine*, 149:708-711.

Brenner, L. H. 1988. Good medicine makes good ethical sense. *Medical Ethics for the Physician*, 3.

Burge, S. K. 1989. Violence against women as a health care issue. *Family Medicine*, 21, 368-73.

Davis, J. E. 1988. National initiatives for care of the medically needy. *Journal of the American Medical Association*, 259.

de Beaufort, I. 1988. *HIV—Infection and AIDS: Some Ethical Questions*. The Netherlands: Institute for Bioethics.

Eisenstein, Z. R. 1988. *The Female Body and the Law*. Berkeley, CA: University of California Press.

Friedman, E. 1988. Women and medicine: From tension to truce. *The Western Journal of Medicine*, 149, 726-28.

Gilligan, C. 1982. *In a Different Voice*. Cambridge, MA: Harvard University Press.

Grande, P. 1990. "Gender gap plagues U.S. health studies." *Cleveland Plain Dealer*, (July 29, 1990).

Morgenthau, H. 1978. *Politics among Nations*, Fifth Edition. New York: Knoft.

New York Times (February 12, 1989).

Nodding, N. 1982. *Caring*. Berkeley, CA: University of California Press.

Payer, L. 1988. *Medicine and Culture*. New York: Penguin Books.

Scully, T. and Scully, C. 1989. *Making Medical Decisions*. New York: Fireside Press.

Women: The road ahead. 1991. *Time* 136 (Special Issue), 66-67.

19

Communicating About Death
By Gary L. Kreps

Introduction

Death is a difficult and uncomfortable subject of discussion for many people, especially for Americans who generally view death as an inappropriate and taboo topic for interpersonal communication (Cassem, 1976; Dumont and Foss, 1972; Lofland, 1978; Mills, Reisler, Robinson, and Vermilye, 1976; Schneidman, 1971). A common communication strategy used in response to talk about death is avoidance, typically operationalized with comments like: "Don't be morbid," or "Can't you talk about something more pleasant" (Dumont and Foss, 1972). Even when the topic of death is not overtly avoided, it is rarely discussed frankly and openly (Patterson, 1976; Raab, 1983). Death-talk is usually quite superficial, where death is either mentioned briefly in passing conversation, discussed reticently in hushed tones, addressed with euphemisms such as "lost," "gone," or "passed away," or minimized with the use of jokes and humor (Davidson, 1976; Gonzalez, 1986, 1987). The ways Americans typically communicate about death clearly illustrate the cultural stigma surrounding death and the process of dying.

The reluctance of Americans to communicate frankly and openly about death is clearly evidenced by the results of a national survey of over 30,000 Americans conducted by Schneidman (1971). In a report of this survey he concludes, "so forbidden has death been in our culture that one-third of the respondents could not recall from childhood a single instance of discussion of death within the family circle. In more than one-third of the families it was mentioned with discomfort, and in only 30% was death talked about openly" (Schneidman, 1971, p. 44). Death is clearly a troublesome topic of conversation for Americans.

The difficulties people have discussing death limits their abilities to use human communication to help make sense of death and dying (Kubler-Ross, 1969). Yet, death is an important, influential, and inevitable life experience that warrants

Reprinted with permission from the *Journal of Communication Theory*, 4 (1988): 2-13.

frank and therapeutic communication. Therapeutic interpersonal communication has the potential to help people cope with difficult life experiences like death and dying (Kreps, 1986; Kreps & Thornton, 1984). The tendency for Americans to avoid open discussion about death minimizes their opportunities to engage in therapeutic communication to help themselves and others cope with the many ambiguities and fears surrounding the phenomenon of death.

Most of the research conducted and literature written about communicating about death has taken a clinical orientation, focusing on the ways in which formal health care providers can communicate therapeutically with terminally ill individuals, with those who survive the deaths of loved ones, and with those people who have pathological fears about death (see: Cassata, 1983; Cassem, 1976; Coombs & Powers, 1975; Gonzalez, 1986, 1987; Kubler-Ross, 1969). Death is an important topic of discussion, not only for health care providers and terminally ill patients, but for all people as a normal part of their everyday lives (Raab, 1983). Recognition of human mortality indicates that all people are in the process of dying from the moment they are born (Parsons, Fox, & Lidz, 1973). All people have to come to grips with death and dying, not just those persons labeled as "terminally ill." Moreover, the current propensity for training formal health care providers (physicians, nurses, therapists, etc.) to communicate about death places health care professionals with the primary responsibility for providing therapeutic communication about death and dying to the public, underscoring the cultural stigma surrounding death-talk and the inability of most people to communicate effectively about death in everyday life.

While the clinical orientation to the study of communication and death is certainly relevant to health care practice (since many health care providers have direct contact with death and dying), it puts much too much responsibility on the health care professions to provide the American public with all necessary therapeutic communication about death. There are far too many Americans who need personal support and feedback about death for health care professionals to possibly be able to reach (Knott, 1979). Furthermore, health care professionals do not have the time nor are they likely to be willing to take on society-wide responsibility for communicating therapeutically about death.

This provider orientation to communicating about death also does little to help the general public learn how to communicate therapeutically about death in everyday life. Death becomes a salient issue for most people when significant others (the people who influence them the most: family, friends, leaders, celebrities, coworkers) face death. Similarly, personal threats to life, such as serious accidents or illnesses, also force people to confront the issues of how to interpret and understand the phenomenon of death, how to prepare and react to death, and how to communicate about death. Making health care providers responsible for death-talk skirts the larger and more relevant issue of communicating about death informally in everyday life, where the vast majority of all therapeutic communication actually occurs (Kreps & Thornton, 1984).

The central argument in this paper is that the personal apprehensions and difficulties in communicating about death that many Americans face pose significant problems for these people. Effective interpersonal communication about death and dying can serve several therapeutic functions for individuals, helping them cope with the many complex issues surrounding human mortality (Cassata, 1983; Mills, Reisler, Robinson, & Vermilye, 1976). This paper will examine several primary reasons why Americans have so much difficulty communicating candidly about death, will identify several prevalent communication strategies used by Americans to talk about death, and will explore the implications of current death communication practices for the provision of therapeutic communication about death and dying in everyday life.

The Complexity of Death and Dying

Death is an extremely pervasive, ubiquitous, and equivocal phenomenon confronting human beings. Death is pervasive because it is relevant to all people. Death is a powerful, relentless phenomenon that has direct influences on all people. There is no way to escape death. Death interrupts all human endeavors. It rarely can be postponed or reversed. The finality of death makes the experience extremely potent. The fact that when significant others die they will not return poses a serious loss for those who care about the persons who have died and have depended upon these people. The pervasiveness of death makes death and the dying process an important and influential topic for interpersonal communication.

Death is ubiquitous because it is such a common phenomenon in society. All people die. During our lifetimes we are likely to encounter the deaths of many different people. Kalish and Reynolds (1976) report there are few people who do not recall having encountered the death and dying of others. Moreover, sooner or later we each must face our own death. Because death is such a prevalent societal phenomenon in human experience it is important for people to be able to talk frankly and openly about death to help prepare for and respond to death and the process of dying.

Death is also an equivocal phenomenon because there are many unanswered questions and mysteries surrounding death. The equivocal nature of death and dying makes it difficult for many people to talk about death and come to grips with the phenomenon. When presented with a situation concerning death most people feel uncomfortable and are unsure of what to say or do (Corr, 1976). Death is an especially complex and equivocal social phenomenon in modern American culture where death is often presented in stereotypic and unrealistic ways. American culture provides few satisfying answers to questions about death like: What happens to us when we die? Why do we die? How and when will we die? How does it feel to die? Difficult questions surrounding the experiences of death and dying certainly outnumber the satisfying societal answers that are available.

The Importance of Communicating About Death

The pervasive and ubiquitous aspects of death make it a major life issue for Americans to examine, confront, and resolve. The equivocal nature of death, however, makes it an extremely difficult topic for many people to discuss. This is a terrible paradox where death is a central human phenomenon that people must confront, yet it is also an issue suffering from significant cultural mystery and stigma that inhibits meaningful communication about death in everyday life.

The very equivocality that makes death a difficult topic to communicate about, may also provide a rationale for why frank, open, and therapeutic communication about death and dying is so very important in everyday life. Weick (1969) suggests that in social organization and adaptation people engage in interpersonal communication patterns (cycles) that help them resolve difficult problems they face that they are not able to handle through routine activities (through rules). Human communication helps people cope with equivocality in their lives by providing them with insight into difficult and challenging social situations, like coping with death and dying. Therapeutic communication about death can help provide communicators with relevant information to help them effectively interpret and respond to the situations confronting them concerning death (Kreps, 1986; Kreps & Thornton, 1984).

American Interpretations of Death and Dying

American culture tends to avoid and deny death, perhaps because the culture encourages people to adopt personal images of self-determination and control, narcissism and instant gratification, as well as youthfulness and vitality that are inconsistent with the reality of death (Guttman, 1973; Howards & Scott, 1971; Mack, 1973). With the exception of suicide or murder, two socially unacceptable strategies for dealing with death, death is rarely a social phenomenon that is under one's personal control. Death is a human experience that directly contradicts the will to live, survive, and prosper, which are primary human goals in American culture. Furthermore, the lifeless nature of physical death is the very antithesis of youthful vitality.

There are many euphemisms commonly used to help people superficially discuss death in American culture. Euphemisms are substitute terms and phrases commonly used in human communication to help people discuss uncomfortable, offensive, or stigmatized topics without mentioning those topics directly. Death euphemisms help disguise and minimize death and the dying process. They help to reduce people's fears about death and make death appear to be less permanent and under more personal control than it actually is (Davidson, 1976).

The most common euphemisms used to communicate about death describe death as a vague active process that is presumably under the control of the dead or dying person. Some of these active process death euphemisms include "passing away," "traveling to the great beyond," "moving to another place," "departed," "going to a better land," "going to kingdom come," "going the way of all flesh," "shuffling off one's mortal coil," "awakening to life immortal," "making one's exit," "going to glory," "buying it," "losing it," "biting the bullet," "kicking the bucket," "going to the last roundup," "taking the last curtain call," "turning in one's chips," "shoving off," "surrendering one's life," or "going to the happy hunting grounds." Death is also routinely euphemized as a vague process that is done to a person, placing the locus of control for death away from the individual and on to some vague external force. Common external locus of control death euphemisms include "taken away," "released," "called home," "launched into eternity," or "in the grasp of the grim reaper." Death is also commonly euphemized as a passive, relaxed process which minimizes discomfort about death and dying. Some of these relaxed death euphemisms include "sleeping," "dreaming," "reposing," "at rest," "resting easy," "borne into a better world," or "out of one's misery." Use of death euphemisms helps people talk about death without openly facing the difficult realities of death and dying, yet they do not help people communicate openly and frankly about their feelings and experiences concerning death and dying.

Death is often presented as either terrifying, horrible, or humorous occurrences in cultural narratives. Typical cultural narratives concerning death and dying are legends and stories recounted within social groups, such as when frightening campfire stories are told to young campers, legends and superstitions about monsters are passed on from generation to generation, or jokes about corpses are shared by medical interns (Gonzalez, 1986, 1987; Hyde, 1985). Horror stories often reinforce unrealistic fears people have about death, while humorous death tales (dark humor) often minimize the pervasiveness of the death phenomenon in modern society and keep people from recognizing the importance of communicating candidly, sensitively, and therapeutically about death.

Death is also presented unrealistically in public communication media such as books, television programs, and films (Peretz, 1976). For example, there is a long-standing genre of horror films based upon death and dying, especially concerning the awakening of the dead. Such films include "Frankenstein," "Dracula," "The Night of the Living Dead," and "The Mummy," where the dead are generally presented as frightening and malevolent monsters to be avoided at all costs. Similarly, there is the all too common film and television artistic convention of having people (usually women) react to the discovery of a dead body with terror, typically screaming in horror and fainting. This artistic convention reinforces the cultural stereotype that death is horrible, frightening, mysterious, and unnatural. Yet, death is a very natural occurrence. Death is no less natural or more mysterious a process than birth, which paradoxically is viewed as a very positive and joyous phenomenon. Most people revel in the mystery of birth. Yet, can you imagine most people reveling in the mystery of death? The ways death is communicated about in American culture, demonstrated through use of death euphemisms, recounting of morbid folklore, use of dark humor, and portrayals of horror stories in mass media, clearly reflects the social stigma surrounding death in society (Choron, 1972). These patterns for communicating about death also reinforce the stigma surrounding death, limit the abilities of Americans to engage in candid communication about death and dying, and also limit the opportunities Americans have for giving and receiving therapeutic communication concerning death.

Conclusions

Avoiding, denying, and minimizing death and dying phenomena serves to exacerbate the difficulties Americans have communicating meaningfully about death by unrealistically representing death and failing to provide people with successful strategies for communicating therapeutically about death and dying. Avoiding discussion about death is used as a symbolic strategy for helping Americans to avoid the inevitability of death. (Out of sight, out of mind.) Yet, avoidance also serves to increase the fears people hold about death. The unfamiliar is always more fearful than the familiar, and the strategy of avoiding communication about death keeps Americans from becoming more familiar with the phenomenon of death. Due to avoidance many people are unprepared to talk about death when faced with the death of a loved one or when faced with their own impending death, severely limiting their ability to seek and utilize social support from others. Moreover, by avoiding communication about death in everyday life many people are unprepared to provide social support to dying individuals or those who are grieving, exacerbating the pain and discomfort of the dying and the grief-stricken. The strategy of avoiding communication about death, while comforting for Americans in the short run, invariably leads to great discomfort for many individuals in the long run.

Educational programs should be developed to help people confront the phenomenon of death (Knott, 1979; Mills, Reisler, Robinson, & Vermilye, 1976; Morgan, 1980). Such programs would encourage individuals to candidly discuss their questions and fears concerning death and dying. Effective educational programs would also provide individuals with strategies for communicating therapeutically with others concerning death, helping these individuals use human communication to demystify the death experience, come to grips with their own mortality, and provide social support to others.

References

Cassata, D. M. 1983. Death and dying: Communication parameters and perspectives. *Journal of Communication Therapy*, 1, 145-54.

Cassem, N. H. 1976. The anatomy of resistance to talking about death and dying. In T. J. Fleming, A. H. Kutscher, D. Peretz, and I. K. Goldberg (eds.), *Communicating issues in thanatology*, 65-70. New York: MSS Information Corporation.

Choron, J. 1972. *Death and modern man.* New York: Collier Books.

Coombs, R. H., and Powers, P. S. 1975. Socialization for death: the physician's role. In L. H. Lofland (ed.), *Toward a sociology of death and dying*, 15-36. Beverly Hills, CA: Sage.

Corr, C. A. 1976. Living with the changing face of death. In H. Wass (ed.), *Dying: Facing the facts*, 44-72. New York: McGraw-Hill.

Davidson, H. A. 1976. The lexicon of death. In T. J. Fleming, A. H. Kutscher, D. Peretz, and I. K. Goldberg (eds.), *Communicating issues in thanatology*, 299-300. New York: MSS Information Corporation.

Dumont, R. G., and Foss, D. C. 1972. *The American view of death: Acceptance or denial.* Cambridge, MA: Schenkman Publishing Company.

Gonzalez, M. 1986. *Communication with patients who are dying: The effects of medical education.* Unpublished doctoral dissertation, University of Texas, Austin.

Gonzalez, M. May, 1987. *We called him "Al": Anatomy lab as model for doctor-patient communication.* Paper presented to the International Communication Association Conference, Montreal, Canada.

Guttman, D. 1973. The premature gerontocracy: Themes of aging and death in the youth culture. In A. Mack (ed.), *Death in American Experience*, 50-82. New York: Schocken Books.

Howards, A., and Scott, R. A. 1971. Cultural values and attitudes toward death. In F. G. Scott and R. M. Brewer (eds.), *Confrontations of death*, 16-25. Corvallis, OR: Continuing Education Publications.

Hyde, M. J. August, 1985. *Medical technology and its dilemmas: Telling stories about life and death.* Paper presented to the Summer Conference on Health Communication, Northwestern University, Evanston, IL.

Kalish, R. A., and Reynolds, D. K. 1976. *Death and ethnicity: A psychocultural study.* Los Angeles: University of Southern California Press.

Knott, J. E. 1979. Death education for all. In H. Wass (ed.), *Dying: Facing the facts*, 385-403. Washington, DC: Hemisphere Books.

Kreps, G. L. 1986. *Organizational communication: Theory and practice.* White Plains, NY: Longman.

Kreps, G. L., and Thornton, B. C. 1984. *Health communication: Theory and practice.* New York: Longman.

Kubler-Ross, E. 1969. *On death and dying.* New York: Macmillan.

Kubler-Ross, E. 1974. *Questions and answers on death and dying.* New York: Macmillan.

Lofland, L. H. 1978. *The craft of dying: The modern face of death.* Beverly Hills, CA: Sage.

Mack, A. (ed.). 1973. *Death in American experience.* New York: Schocken Books.

Mills, G. C., Reisler, R. Jr., Robinson, A. E., and Vermilye, G. 1976. *Discussing death: A guide to death education.* Homewood, IL: ETC Publications.

Morgan, E. 1980. *A manual of death education and simple burial.* Burnsville, NC: Celo Press.

Parsons, T., Fox, R. C., and Lidz, V. M. 1973. The "gift of life" and its reciprocation. In A. Mack (ed.), *Death in American Experience*, 1-49. New York: Schocken Books.

Patterson, P. R. 1976. Society's communication of death to children. In T. J. Fleming, A. H. Kutscher, D. Peretz, and I. K. Goldberg (eds.), *Communicating issues in thanatology,* 205-207. New York: MSS Information Corporation.

Peretz, D. 1976. Television: Violence and the fears of death. In T. J. Fleming, A. H. Kutscher, D. Peretz, and I. K. Goldberg (eds.), *Communicating issues in thanatology,* 201-204. New York: MSS Information Corporation.

Raab, R. A. 1983. *Coping with Death* (rev.ed.). New York: Rosen Publishing Group.

Schneidman, E. 1971. You and death, *Psychology Today,* 5:43-45, 74-80.

Weick, K. 1969. *The social psychology of organizing.* Reading, MA: Addison-Wesley.

Communication and Health Promotion

Communication performs an extremely important role in promoting public health by disseminating relevant health information to the public. Persuasive health communication campaigns can provide individuals with both rationale and direction for adopting health-promoting behaviors. However, the health communication process is deceivingly complex. It is oversimplistic to assume that mere exposure to relevant health information will lead directly to changes in habitual health behaviors. Health-behavior change is a complex process involving many factors, such as the nature of the health behavior to be changed, the individual characteristics of the audience members targeted, and the communication strategies used to reach the audience. Therefore, health communication campaigns must be carefully designed and executed to accomplish their health promotion goals.

Effective health promotion campaigns must be tailored to the specific needs and communication characteristics of target audiences. Audience analysis can provide campaign planners with relevant information about target audiences for designing effective campaigns. Audience segmentation strategies enable the campaign planner to focus health communication efforts on specific and homogenous target audiences that are likely to respond positively to campaign messages. A social marketing perspective to health promotion where campaign messages are seen as products to be tailored to specific audiences (customers) can be effective at achieving campaign goals. It is also advantageous to use powerful theories of human behavior to guide message strategies. Communication channels must be selected that can reach, get the attention of, and influence target audiences. Moreover, evaluation research can provide campaign planners with both formative and summative data about the effectiveness of health promotion strategies.

This section of the book examines the role of communication in health promotion campaigns. The first reading, written specifically for this book by Edward Maibach, examines the uses of behavioral theory to develop AIDS information and health risk prevention campaigns. This reading clearly describes the applications of relevant theory to plan health promotion campaigns strategically. This reading also illustrates why good theory is particularly useful in developing strategies for addressing complex social issues, such as the prevention of AIDS transmission. Maibach describes the use of Bandura's social cognitive theory in public efforts to change health behaviors. He describes how the theory is used to design campaign messages that can enhance the self-efficacy of target audiences to engage in health risk prevention behaviors.

The second reading, written by Craig Lefebvre and June Flora, originally published as a journal article in *Health Education Quarterly*, provides an excellent examination of the use of social marketing in health promotion, describing how specific social marketing principles are applied to the development and implementation of health promotion campaigns. To illustrate social marketing in action, they describe two important communication campaigns that they have worked with, the Pawtucket Heart Health Program "Know Your Cholesterol" campaign and the Stanford Five-City Project Smoker's Challenge II campaign. This reading provides a clear description of the applications of social marketing principles to persuasion and public health promotion.

20

The Use of Behavioral Theory in the Development of AIDS Information Campaigns

By Edward Maibach

AIDS is one of the most pressing health problems in America and the world today, and is likely to remain so into the next century (Hulley & Hearst, 1989). The World Health Organization estimates that 10 million people are currently infected with the AIDS virus. If the epidemic continues unchecked, more than 20 million people worldwide will be infected by the end of this decade. AIDS is a fatal disease; there is no vaccination or cure. Prevention is currently the only method available to curtail the epidemic.

AIDS is an extremely complex disease syndrome, although the mechanisms of its transmission are quite simple. AIDS is transmitted through the exchange of certain bodily fluids including blood, semen, and vaginal secretions. This exchange of these bodily fluids occurs almost exclusively during two activities: (1) sexual intercourse and oral-genital contact; and (2) sharing needles to inject intravenous (IV) drugs. Abstinence from sex and IV drug use can reliably prevent the transmission of the AIDS virus. However, abstinence is often not an acceptable alternative for many people. Fortunately, the risk of exposure can be reduced through other means as well. IV drug users can sterilize their "works" by using bleach and water to clean their needles and syringes. "Safer sex" activities that do not involve the exchange of bodily fluids can be substituted for unsafe sexual activities. This commonly entails the proper use of a latex condom during sexual contact with people who may have been exposed to the AIDS virus.

In general, the American public is quite knowledgeable about the mechanisms of AIDS transmission (Hardy & Dawson, 1989). In some cases, AIDS risk behaviors have begun to change as well. Many homosexuals (Ekstrand & Coates, 1990), heterosexuals (Maibach, 1990) and IV drug users (Guydish et al., 1990) have responded to the threat of AIDS by modifying their risk

This article was written especially for this collection. Dr. Maibach is a member of the faculty of the School of Public Health at Emory University where he conducts health communication research.

behaviors. However, there are still a large number of Americans who practice behaviors that put them at risk for exposure to the AIDS virus (Baldwin & Baldwin, 1988; Reinisch et al., 1988). In order to make further progress against the epidemic, effective health communication campaigns must be developed to address the needs of people currently engaging in AIDS risk behaviors.

Media and the Fight Against AIDS

Health information campaigns are an important component of public health education (Flora, Maibach & Maccoby, 1989). Information campaigns may be particularly important in the fight against AIDS in that, unlike some public health problems, AIDS risk behaviors are almost exclusively discretionary. People choose to engage in the behaviors that place them at risk; likewise, they can be taught and motivated to enact preventive behaviors instead (Solomon & DeJong, 1989; Kelly et al., 1989).

Federal, state and city health departments, and a variety of foundations and other nonprofit health agencies currently develop AIDS information campaigns to promote AIDS prevention and a variety of other outcomes. For example, the National AIDS Information and Education Program conducted by the U.S. Centers for Disease Control has mounted an intensive television and print media campaign over the past several years. There is, however, little published information regarding the effectiveness of this and other campaign efforts.

Behavioral and communication theory are known to play an important role in the development of effective information campaigns (Rogers & Storey, 1987; Rice & Atkin, 1989). The role of theory in campaign development is even more critical in the absence of evaluation data to indicate what is and is not working. Behavioral theory can provide insight into why people engage in certain behaviors and fail to enact others. Likewise, communication theory can both inform persuasive message development efforts and guide the selection of communication channels to ensure maximal reach within the target audience. AIDS campaigns will be more effective to the extent that such theories are applied during the development and implementation of campaign activities.

Social Cognitive Theory and the Development of AIDS Media

Social cognitive theory (Bandura, 1986) is an excellent theory of both health behavior (Bandura, 1989, 1990a) and mass media effectiveness (Bandura, 1990b). Social cognitive theory (SCT) offers a comprehensive and powerful set of behavior change principles from which to develop health educational media. As a theory of behavior, social cognitive theory has achieved the highest standards of utility, in that it can predict behavior, it can explain behavior, and most importantly, it can be used to help correct dysfunctional behaviors. Moreover, the causal mechanisms specified in social cognitive theory have been shown to operate across a broad spectrum of both health and nonhealth related behaviors. SCT has been used effectively to explain and correct a diverse set of health problems including smoking, weight and dietary control, lack of exercise, failures in contraceptive practices, and AIDS risk behaviors (for recent reviews see Strecher et al., 1986; Bandura, 1990a).

This chapter will briefly discuss and illustrate the implications of SCT for the development of AIDS information campaigns. For the sake of brevity, the discussion will be limited in a number of ways. Only the most cursory description of SCT will be presented. Interested readers should consult other sources for a full description (Bandura, 1986). Although AIDS campaigns can validly have numerous objectives, this chapter will consider only one possible objective, the promotion of condom use. Although information campaigns generally utilize multiple channels of communication, the current discussion will be most relevant to televised media, including video and broadcast television.

AIDS risk reduction recommendations are not terribly complicated, but they can be quite difficult to implement. People need certain skills in order to implement the recommended behaviors. For example, in order to use condoms as a reliable means of reducing AIDS risk, a person must be able to: (1) buy condoms and appropriate lubricants; (2) use condoms properly; (3) have condoms available when they are needed; (4) discuss safe sex before engaging in sexual intercourse, and when appropriate, suggest and insist that condoms be used and used properly; and (5) overcome a partner's resistance to the use of a condom. Some of these skills, such as buying condoms, are not difficult for most people. Others, such as overcoming a partner's resistance to using condoms, can be quite difficult for most people. The first lesson from SCT is that people's confidence in their ability to use their skills (in SCT terminology, their self-efficacy) is the most important predictor of their willingness and ability to do so. An understanding of self-efficacy is necessary to better understand how to promote the development and application of AIDS prevention skills.

Self-efficacy and the promotion of behavior

Self-efficacy is the pivotal concept in SCT in that it mediates between what people know and what they actually apply. Self-efficacy is defined as people's belief in their capabilities to achieve different levels of performance attainment (Bandura, 1977). Success in most areas of human endeavor requires commitment, resourcefulness, and perseverance. These are precisely the qualities addressed by self-efficacy. People's confidence in their ability to overcome the difficulties that are inherent in achieving a behavior are expressed in their assessments of self-efficacy. Self-efficacy is a personal assessment of ability to enact a particular type of behavior under specified conditions.

The importance of self-efficacy can best be understood by a description of its consequences. A person with a strong sense of self-efficacy for a behavior will exhibit a number of characteristics that are conducive to its successful enactment (Bandura, 1986). These characteristics generally include (1) a decision to at least try the behavior; (2) setting a goal for how well or how often the behavior will be performed, and feeling a sense of commitment to that goal; (3) perseverant effort to attain the goal; (4) the use of a variety of goal attainment strategies; (5) the use of analytical problem-solving skills to resolve problems that block goal attainment; (6) interpreting (inevitable) failures as temporary setbacks that have resulted from insufficient effort; and (7) bouncing back quickly from failed efforts. People with little perceived self-efficacy for a behavior typically fail to use these approaches, and consequently, they are generally not successful in enacting the behavior in question.

Most people experience a wide range of self-efficacy expectations, from very low to very high, depending on the behavior being assessed. Self-efficacy expectations, or perceptions of self-efficacy can change over time. Temporal variations in self-efficacy are the result of the way in which perceptions of efficacy are formed. Several types of information influence perceptions of self-efficacy. The availability of these forms of efficacy information can change over time, resulting in concomitant changes in perceptions of efficacy.

Perceived self-efficacy to engage in a behavior is a function of four types of information: (1) previous experience with the behavior or a similar behavior; (2) vicarious experience with the behavior as communicated through live or mediated modeling; (3) verbal persuasion regarding capabilities to engage in the behavior; and (4) inferences from the physiological states that are experienced when anticipating or engaging in the behavior. The importance of each of these sources of information may vary depending on the other sources of efficacy information and a variety of other factors. For example, people can pay more or less attention to any one of the sources of efficacy information at any point in time, thereby influencing their resulting efficacy assessment.

The dynamics of self-efficacy and its causal link to behavior present two major implications for effective AIDS information campaigns. First, because of the causal relationship between self-efficacy and behavior, campaigns that seek to change AIDS prevention behaviors must do so, at least in part, by promoting enhancements in AIDS prevention self-efficacy. AIDS risk behaviors will decrease to the extent that the target audience's perceptions of self-efficacy are enhanced. Secondly, AIDS information campaigns can promote enhancements in AIDS prevention self-efficacy by modeling appropriate AIDS preventive behaviors, thereby supplying viewers with additional vicarious efficacy information. Learning through vicarious experience in this fashion, called observational learning, is another important concept from SCT.

Observational learning and the promotion of self-efficacy

Observational learning is the vicarious acquisition of knowledge from the social environment (Bandura, 1986). The prevalence and importance of observational learning cannot be understated. People learn by watching others. Observational learning is a primary source of both cognitive, affective, and behavioral development. By watching others model unique behaviors, people gather information that allows them to extend their own horizons. This modeled information can include new values, attitudes, emotional reactions, and social, behavioral, and cognitive skills. More importantly, through observation people can also learn the rules for combining thoughts and actions to cope with novel situations.

One of the ways that observational learning influences subsequent behavior is through the promotion of self-efficacy. As noted above, vicarious experience with a behavior through live or mediated modeling is one source of self-efficacy information. When people watch others engage in a behavior, they infer things about their own ability. However, various characteristics of the model, the behavior being modeled, and the modeling situation affect viewers' ability to make inferences about their own ability. For example, people feel more efficacious to the extent that they judge themselves to be as capable as, or more capable than the model. A more complete presentation of the observational learning process is required to elucidate the qualities of effective modeling presentations.

The effectiveness of observational learning is governed by a set of subprocesses: attention, retention, production, and motivation (Bandura, 1986). Each of these will be considered for its relevance to the promotion of self-efficacy and behavior change using AIDS information campaigns.

Implications from the Attentional Subprocess of Observational Learning

There are a multitude of modeling influences in the information environment. The abundance of modeling information is so great that people are able to process only a small part of what is available. People must be selective in choosing which modeling influences to attend to. Only those modeled activities that are attended to are of any value in changing behavior.

Certain properties of modeled activities influence the rate at which people attend to them (see Bandura, 1986; Perry & Furukawa, 1986; Decker & Nathan, 1985; Hosford & Mills, 1983 for detailed discussions of these and subsequent qualities of effective modeling). Unique acts of modeling are more likely to be attended to than are common acts. There is little reason to attend to common events because they offer only a limited amount of new information. Modeling that has functional value to the observer will be attended to more closely than modeling with no obvious value. People pay more attention to the extent that they realize the information is relevant to them. Simple behaviors are more likely to be attended to, and comprehended, than are overly complex acts of modeling. When the modeled behavior is complex in nature, breaking it down into its component parts can help maintain the observer's attention.

Characteristics of the models also influence the degree to which viewers pay attention to acts of modeling. Viewers pay more attention to models who are similar to themselves in terms of age, race, and attitude. Attractive and interesting models are attended to more closely than are unattractive and uninteresting models. Similarly, models who are slightly more socially prestigious than viewers command more of the viewers' attention than do models who are either less prestigious, or considerably more prestigious. Models should be somewhat warm and nurturing in personality rather than strident or uncaring. Models should be somewhat more competent than the viewers at the behavior being modeled, but not too much more competent. If overly competent models are shown, viewers will be less able to relate to them, and will infer less about their own ability to engage in the behavior being modeled. A variety of different models should be portrayed, in that any one model may or may not command the attention of a potential audience member. Using a number of different models will maximize the proportion of the audience who actually do pay attention. And similarly, having the models demonstrate their behavior in a variety of different settings will be more effective than behavioral demonstrations that are limited in setting. In order to gain and hold the attention of the target audience, AIDS campaigns must follow these guidelines in selecting appropriate models to demonstrate the skills necessary to engage in risk reduction.

Implications from the Retentional Subprocess of Observational Learning

Memory is a major barrier between observing an act of modeling and being able to reproduce what was observed. The retentional subprocess addresses this barrier. People remember complex information only to the extent that they have organized it into a form that is easily recalled. People often fail to process information sufficiently for subsequent use when they are merely passive observers. There are two ways to improve viewers' retention of information. The first method is to encourage observers to actively process the modeled information. This can be done by having them create either verbal representations of what they have seen or by having them create vivid visual imagery that will help them to remember the information.

Second, the act of modeling itself can be organized in ways that help viewers process and retain the information. Rather than simply demonstrating a behavior, models can explain the rules they use to guide their behavior. Most AIDS prevention skills have an important cognitive component. This cognitive component of modeling is generally unobservable to viewers unless it is somehow made observable. By revealing that which is normally not observable (for example, the model's thought process while negotiating with a potential partner about having sex), viewers will better understand the requirements of a successful performance. Models should contrast effective with ineffective behavior. Viewers are better prepared to the extent that they understand what works as well as what does not work. Complex behaviors should be made to seem less complex to the viewer. This can be done by breaking a complex behavior down into its component parts. Models can isolate and demonstrate each of the component parts of a complex behavior one at a time. They can then demonstrate how to combine the component parts into the larger behavior. For example, successfully dispelling a potential partner's unwillingness to talk about safe sex may have certain discreet elements. Each of these elements should be demonstrated, as well as how to put them all together. Finally, diverse and creative ways to engage in the behavior should be modeled. This will help viewers to identify how to adapt the skills they have seen performed in new situations and to create novel approaches to the behavior.

Implications from the Production Subprocess of Observational Learning

Learning and ability to reproduce are not necessarily synonymous. People can learn new behaviors observationally before they are able to enact them. The production subprocess is where people attempt to reproduce the behaviors or cognitive skills that they have learned observationally. By engaging in a trial behavior, people sometimes find that their conception of the behavior isn't complete enough to allow them to perform it properly. The feedback that they receive during a trial behavior can help them to identify their performance strengths and weaknesses, and thereby aid in refining subsequent performances.

To enhance observational learning, viewers should be encouraged to rehearse what they have seen. Behavioral rehearsal is known to be an extremely effective means of enhancing self-efficacy. Either a trial behavior or a low-level version of the behavior can be recommended. For example, audience members can be encouraged to speak with their friends about AIDS prevention as a warm-up to speaking with a sex partner. Campaign messages can also prompt viewers to imagine themselves enacting the behavior. This type of cognitive rehearsal has been shown to be effective in enhancing viewers' perceptions of AIDS prevention self-efficacy (Maibach, 1990). Rehearsal of any type is especially effective when instructive feedback is provided to help guide the development of skills and efficacy. However, information campaigns have few obvious means of providing instructive feedback to audience members. "Feed forward," or diagnostic information given in advance, is one possible way of approximating the effects of feedback with campaign messages.

Implications from the Motivational Subprocess of Observational Learning

SCT distinguishes between the acquisition and performance of behaviors. People can learn a behavior or cognitive skill without being motivated to enact what they learned. Self-efficacy plays a large role in motivation. Outcome expectations and incentives also play a major role in motivating behavioral enactments. Each of these will be considered in turn.

People are generally motivated to perform behaviors for which they feel highly efficacious. Conversely, people tend not to be able to sustain much motivation for activities at which they feel inefficacious. Therefore, one of the most effective ways of promoting motivation for a behavior is by enhancing people's sense of self-efficacy associated with that behavior. Self-efficacy can be enhanced with appropriate use of behavioral modeling.

Motivation to enact a behavior is also influenced by people's expectations that doing so will produce positive consequences. In social cognitive theory, these are called outcome expectations (Bandura, 1986). Given a minimum level of self-efficacy, the more positive a person's outcome expectations, the more motivated they should be to enact the behavior. However, there are often many relevant outcomes associated with any behavior. For example, a few outcomes that may be associated with condom use include disease prevention, sexual gratification, interpersonal satisfaction, and peer acceptance. Some of these outcomes may be perceived to be at odds with other outcomes.

If members of the target audience believe that a recommended AIDS prevention behavior creates negative consequences, the campaign must identify ways to enact the behavior that avoid the negative consequences of concern. For example, a sizable portion of women in the target audience may believe that condoms will protect them from AIDS and other sexually transmitted diseases, but they may also believe that condoms detract from their partner's sexual pleasure, and that they risk alienating a prospective partner by raising the issue of condoms. While these concerns may be valid in some cases, they are groundless in many others. Campaign messages must be developed to address these concerns. Either a factual approach or a modeling approach can be taken to convey the fact that wearing condoms does not have to interfere with sexual pleasure, and that talking to prospective partners can enhance rather than jeopardize a relationship.

The final contribution to motivation comes in the form of the incentives that are associated with the behavior. There are three classes of incentives that can motivate behavior. These include direct incentives, vicarious incentives and self-produced incentives. Each of these can exert a powerful influence.

Direct incentives refer to the economic gains that will result from engaging in the behavior. Such gains can include money and other material goods, social status, or any form of direct pleasure associated with performance of the behavior. However, most behaviors do not lead directly to gain. More typically, people engage in activities that they anticipate will pay off in the long run. The incentives are vicarious in that they are based in anticipation of future gain as a result of having observed other people being rewarded for successful performance of the behavior. Self-incentives are those incentives that are developed and provided solely by the self. There are two types of self-incentives: tangible and self-evaluative. Tangible self-incentives are self-provided rewards for performance of a behavior. These can take a variety of forms including material rewards (e.g., new clothes), sensory rewards (e.g., a special meal), and activity rewards (e.g., taking time off work). The second type of self-incentive, self-evaluations, offers nothing of tangible value but can be extremely motivating. People can exhibit extreme perseverance in their actions when they are following their principles or in pursuit of personal excellence. Such behavior cannot readily be explained by direct or vicarious incentives. The active pursuit of and progress toward personal goals causes people to feel good about themselves. Feeling good about oneself, feeling challenged, and feeling self-empowered can provide a powerful source of motivation.

Although AIDS campaigns cannot actually provide incentives for behavior, they can portray the incentives, and thereby make them more salient. For example, a tangible incentive associated with the use of a condom is the prevention of disease transmission (and possibly unwanted pregnancy). A vicarious incentive might be the development of a stronger relationship in response to an open discussion about the need for sexual precautions. A self-evaluative incentive might simply be people feeling good about themselves for doing the right thing. Although these three examples are not necessarily accurate or appropriate, incentives that will motivate the target audience to avoid unsafe sex practices can creatively be presented in campaign materials.

Conclusion

AIDS campaigns can be developed to reduce the prevalence of AIDS risk behaviors. The American public is well aware that the AIDS virus is transmitted sexually and through the sharing of needles for IV drug use. Campaign materials must now identify and demonstrate the skills that people need to reduce their risk. The principles of observational learning should be employed in the development of campaign messages. These messages should attempt to enhance self-efficacy, promote a positive outcome expectation, and encourage continued motivation to avoid AIDS risk practices. Cognitive skills (how the models think about safer sex), affective skills (how the models feel about safer sex), and behavioral skills (how the models actually arrange their lives so that they can avoid unsafe sex) must all be made explicit.

This discussion has briefly covered only one aspect of campaign design: the use of behavioral theory in the design of campaign messages. Successful campaign efforts require considerable attention to a large number of factors including identification of the target audience, selection of appropriate channels of communication, and application of formative, process and summative evaluation techniques (Lefebvre & Flora, 1988). A number of excellent resources are available to the reader interested in learning more about the communication campaign process (e.g., Rogers & Storey, 1987; Rice & Atkin, 1989; Salmon, 1989; Kotler & Roberto, 1989).

References

Baldwin, J. D. & Baldwin, J. I. 1988. Factors affecting AIDS-related sexual risk-taking behavior among college students. *The Journal of Sex Research* 25, 181-96.

Bandura, A. 1977. Self-efficacy: Toward a unified theory of behavioral change. *Psychological Review* 84, 191-215.

Bandura, A. 1986. *Social foundations of thought and action: A social cognitive approach.* Englewood Cliffs, NJ: Prentice Hall.

Bandura, A. 1989. Perceived self-efficacy in the exercise of control over AIDS infection. In V. Mays, G. Albee and S. Schneider (eds.), *Primary prevention of AIDS: Psychological approaches.* (pp. 128-41) Newbury Park, CA: Sage.

Bandura, A. 1990a. Self-efficacy mechanism in physiological activation and health-promoting behavior. In J. Madden, S. Matthysse and J. Barchas (eds.), *Adaptation, learning and affect.* In press. New York: Raven Press.

Bandura, A. 1990b. Social cognitive theory of mass communication. In J. Groebel and P. Winterhoff (eds.), *Empirische medienpsychologie.* In press. Munich: Psychologie Verlags Union.

Decker, P. & Nathan, B. 1985. *Behavioral modeling training: Principles and applications.* New York: Praeger.

Ekstrand, M. & Coates, T. 1990. Maintenance of safer sexual behaviors and predictors of risky sex: The San Francisco Men's Health Study. *American Journal of Public Health* 80, 973-77.

Flora, J., Maibach, E. & Maccoby, N. 1989. The role of mass media across four levels of health promotion intervention. *Annual Review of Public Health* 10:181-201.

Guydish, J., Abramowitz, A., Woods, W., Black, D. & Sorenson, J. 1990. Changes in needle sharing behavior among intravenous drug users: San Francisco, 1986-88. *American Journal of Public Health* 80, 995-97.

Hardy, A. & Dawson, D. 1989. AIDS knowledge and attitudes for October and November 1988. National Center for Health Statistics-Advance data No.167.

Hosford, R. & Mills, M. 1983. Video in social skills training. In P. Dowrick and S. Biggs (eds.), *Using video: Psychological and social applications* (pp. 125-50). New York: Wiley.

Hulley, S. & Hearst, N. 1989. The worldwide epidemiology and prevention of AIDS. In V. Mays, G. Albee and S. Schneider (eds.), *Primary prevention of AIDS: Psychological approaches* (pp. 47-71). Newbury Park, CA: Sage.

Kelly, J. A., St. Lawrence, J., Hood, H. & Brasfield, T. 1989. Behavioral intervention to reduce AIDS risk activities. *Journal of Consulting and Clinical Psychology* 57, 60-67.

Kotler, P. & Roberto, E. 1989. *Social marketing: Strategies for changing public behavior.* New York: Free Press.

Lefebvre, R. C. & Flora, J. A. 1988. Social marketing and public health intervention. *Health Education Quarterly* 15:299-315.

Maibach, E. 1990. Symbolic Modeling and Cognitive Rehearsal: Using Video to Promote Safer Sex. Unpublished doctoral dissertation. Stanford University.

Perry, M. & Furukawa, M. J. 1986. Modeling methods. In F. Kanfer and A. Goldstein (eds.) *Helping people change,* Third Edition, (pp. 66-110). New York: Pergamon.

Reinisch, J. M., Sanders, S. & Ziemba-Davis, M. 1988. The study of sexual behavior in relation to the transmission of human immunodeficiency virus: Caveats and recommendations. *American Psychologist* 43, 921-27.

Rice, R. & Atkin, C. 1989. *Public communication campaigns,* Second Edition. Newbury Park, CA: Sage.

Rogers, E. & Storey, D. 1987. Communication campaigns. In C. Berger and S. Chaffee (eds.), *Handbook of communication science* (pp. 817-46). Newbury Park, CA: Sage.

Salmon, C. T. 1989. *Information campaigns: Balancing social values and social change.* Newbury Park, CA: Sage.

Solomon, M. & DeJong, W. 1989. Preventing AIDS and other STD's through condom promotion: A patient education intervention. *American Journal of Public Health* 79, 453-58.

Strecher, V., DeVellis, B., Becker, M. & Rosenstock, I. M. 1986. The role of self-efficacy in achieving health behavior change. *Health Education Quarterly* 13, 73-91.

21

Social Marketing and Public Health Intervention

By R. Craig Lefebvre and June A. Flora

The rapid proliferation of community-based health education programs has outpaced the knowledge base of behavior change strategies that are appropriate and effective for public health interventions. However, experiences from a variety of large-scale studies suggest that principles and techniques of social marketing may help bridge this gap. This article discusses eight essential aspects of the social marketing process: the use of a consumer orientation to develop and market intervention techniques, exchange theory as a model from which to conceptualize service delivery and program participation, audience analysis and segmentation strategies, the use of formative research in program design and pretesting of intervention materials, channel analysis for devising distribution systems and promotional campaigns, employment of the "marketing mix" concept in intervention planning and implementation, development of a process tracking system, and a management process of problem analysis, planning, implementation, feedback and control functions. Attention to such variables could result in more cost-effective programs that reach larger numbers of the target audience.

Social Marketing and Public Health Intervention

Experiences gleaned from The National High Blood Pressure Education Program,[1] the Stanford Three-Community Study,[2] and other public health education efforts have pointed to the usefulness of social marketing principles in formulating and implementing broad-based behavior change programs. The expansion of health promotion/education activities from those that focus primarily on individuals and small groups to those that target whole communities, segments of society, or entire populations has brought with it the

Reprinted by permission of John Wiley and Sons, Inc. from *Health Education Quarterly*, 15 (1988): 299-315, Copyright © 1988. Dr. Lefebvre is director of Intervention Services at Prospect Associates in Rockville, Maryland. Dr. Flora is a member of the faculty of the Department of Communication at Stanford University.

realization that traditional methods may not be as applicable or effective in these larger contexts. As practitioners gain more experience in working for health-promotive changes in populations, the shortcomings of classic educational approaches — especially group-based models in stimulating changes in behavior — have become apparent. Recent analyses of participant data from a large cardiovascular disease prevention program have shown, for instance, that less than 20% of all contacts have been made through group methods of behavior change. In addition, it was found that over 90% of weight loss and exercise group participants were female and came from highly specific age groups (i.e., younger to middle-aged).[3] These data underscore three major problems which have confronted intervention efforts and stimulated the search for new methods to alter a population's health practices:

1. the limited reach of individual counseling and small group programming;
2. the low penetration of individual or group-based health education methods in many segments of the population, especially "hard-to-reach" groups; and
3. the overwhelming nature of the task to develop programs that will effect changes in populations, given the limited resources that are usually available and the lack of appropriate technology development.

This article reviews basic social marketing principles, techniques and their application. The discussion is based on the authors' experiences in two large community-based projects — the Pawtucket Heart Health Program[4] (PHHP) and The Stanford Five-City Project[5] — from which examples will be presented. The challenges posed by these projects lead us to conclude that social marketing is an invaluable referent from which to design, implement, evaluate, and manage large-scale, broad-based, behavior-change focused programs.

Social Marketing: A Definition

Many authors have offered definitions of social marketing. They usually include the notion that social marketing involves increasing the acceptability of ideas or practices in a target group,[6] that it is a process for solving problems,[7] that it applies marketing thoughts to the introduction and dissemination of ideas and issues,[8] and that it is a strategy for translating scientific knowledge into effective education programs (i.e., developing effective communication strategies).[9] Social marketing concepts and methods borrow heavily from the traditional marketing literature. However, social marketing is distinguished by its emphasis on so-called "nontangible" products — ideas, attitudes, lifestyle changes — as opposed to the more tangible products and services that are the focus of marketing in the business, health-care and nonprofit service sectors. While this lack of tangible goods and services is cited as a challenge to social marketers, we will provide examples of how tangible products and services can be developed and employed to support social marketing efforts. It should also be noted that often the business marketing and social marketing distinction can be blurred, as when fast service restaurants promote the nutritional value of their products, breakfast food manufacturers advertise the risk reducing qualities of their products, or condom manufacturers provide information on AIDS. It is often necessary to identify the objective of the source to clarify the issue of whether one is interested in increasing market share versus improving the public health. The two are not necessarily exclusive, yet expressed social concern can often times mask more "bottom-line" interests.

Social marketing principles are especially well-suited for the task of translating necessarily complex educational messages and behavior change techniques into concepts and products that will be received and acted upon by a large segment of the population. Brief social marketing campaigns cannot be expected to result in substantial cognitive and/or behavior changes; yet, their strategic and continuous application are viewed here as a necessary condition for effective public health interventions.

We have distilled the essential aspects of social marketing into eight components: (1) a consumer orientation to realize organizational goals, (2) an emphasis on voluntary exchanges of goods and services between providers and consumers, (3) research in audience analysis and segmentation strategies, (4) the use of formative research in product or message design and the pretesting of these materials, (5) an analysis of distribution (or communication) channels, (6) use of the "marketing mix" — that is, utilizing and blending product, price, place, and promotion characteristics in intervention planning and implementation, (7) a process tracking system with both integrative and control functions, and (8) a management process that involves problem analysis, planning, implementation and feedback functions. Each of these components will be discussed with particular reference to the field of public health intervention/education.

Consumer Orientation

Social marketing has evolved from business marketing practices — the analysis by Kotler and Zaltman[10] marked its emergence as a distinct discipline. Business marketing practice in turn has evolved through a series of stages to its present-day consumer orientation.[6]

A "production orientation," the predominant business attitude for the first half of this century, is characterized by a concern for increasing output and reducing costs. In health promotion an analog would be "more programs at less cost" for the client, but more so for the sponsoring agency. The "we know what's good for them" attitude of health professionals toward their target groups dramatizes this approach.

The second phase of business philosophy, a "sales orientation," has been typified by a selling and promotion effort directed toward generating high sales and high profits. Social advertising methods that rely upon promotion to "sell" products, such as exercise equipment and "quit smoking" programs, are examples of this approach to health education.

Both the production and sales orientations are agency-centered; the generation or sale of the product — whether it be goods, services or ideas — is the goal of the sponsoring organization. Fine[8] has also referred to these types of orientations as "push" marketing, where the agency "pushes" its ideas, products and/or services onto consumers. These approaches give little attention to consumers' needs or preferences in the design or promotion of these products. The role of the client is to buy, or be persuaded to buy, the product. Although in many cases the client cost may not be monetary, as we will see later, all health promotion efforts involve costs to the consumer — costs that the sales approach attempts to convince the consumer he/she should incur.

In contrast to the production and sales orientation, modern business marketing addresses the client's needs and interest in the development and promotion of products and services, or what Fine[8] calls "pull" marketing where consumer's "pull" certain ideas, products and/or services out of agencies. The marketing concept has been defined as (1) a consumers' needs orientation backed by (2) integrated marketing aimed at (3) generating consumer satisfaction as the key to (4) satisfying organizational goals.[5] In the context of public health intervention, this definition can be stated as:

> "Health marketing" refers to health promotion programs that are developed
> to satisfy consumer needs, strategized to reach as broad an audience as
> is in need of the program, and thereby enhance the organization's ability
> to effect population-wide changes in targeted risk behaviors.

As opposed to being "product-driven" (or "expert-driven" — e.g. "we know what they need"), the marketing philosophy underscores the necessity for health agencies to be aware of and responsive to consumer needs. While specific initiatives may be launched by public health professionals in response to data or conditions of which the general populace may not be sufficiently aware (e.g., The National Cholesterol Education Program, results of specific community needs analyses), these efforts should be designed in response to audience needs (i.e., what do they not know?), implemented to meet those needs, effective in satisfying the needs, and monitored both to ensure that they continue to meet these needs and to alert the agency to new or changing needs in the target group. A consumer orientation does not stop at the needs assessment stage. Rather, through the process of concept development and materials production, consumer input is sought and utilized by the developers. Knowing that "cholesterol awareness" is a need is not enough. One must also ensure that the products and services designed to meet this need will be attended to, comprehended, and acted upon by the target group.

A number of obstacles hinder the adoption and maintenance of a consumer orientation in public health oriented agencies. These barriers include (1) a lack of clearly specified organizational objectives (or mission), owing to a lack of intra-organizational consensus and/or inadequate audience needs assessment, (2) a failure to identify key target audiences which undermines valid needs surveys, (3) community organization pressures that place territorial/professional objectives above consumer needs, (4) organizational biases that favor "expert-driven" programs, and (5) situations that require working with multiple intermediaries who, in turn, may modify and dilute the message before it reaches the consumer. Recognition of these barriers from the outset of program planning, and the development of strategies that specifically address each of them, will help insure that consumer needs are solicited, listened to, and acted upon by the responsible agency.

Exchange Theory

While the underlying philosophy of marketing can be described as being consumer-driven, the primary operational mechanism is based on exchange theory.[6] According to exchange theory, individuals, groups, or organizations have resources that they want to exchange, or might conceivably exchange, for perceived benefits. In this sense, many different types of transactions could be characterized as exchanges. However, to be considered marketing transactions, ideas, products or services must be deliberately introduced into the transaction with a buy-and-sell intention. Such transactions include such diverse processes as information dissemination, public relations, lobbying efforts, and advocacy causes.[8]

Exchanges can occur on a number of levels: people can be threatened to exchange ("Eat cheese or die"), they can be coerced to exchange ("Just one more time — please?"), they can be commanded to exchange ("Uncle Sam wants *you!*"), or they can choose to exchange voluntarily. Marketing approaches focus on facilitating the voluntary exchange of resources. This needs to be distinguished from what many people mistakenly perceive as marketing; that is, product advertising which preempts voluntary choice, i.e., "high pressure sales." The critical difference between marketing and other forms of persuasion lies in marketing's orientation toward satisfying consumer interests through the utilization of techniques that facilitate *voluntary* exchanges between the consumer and the producer.

People have many resources available to them for exchange. In health promotion, the most important include money, time, physical and cognitive effort (such as is needed to maintain an exercise program or quit smoking), lifestyle, psychological factors (e.g., coping skills/abilities, self-efficacy/esteem) and social contacts. Resources typically available in health agencies include money, technical expertise, and a variety of ideas, products, and services. While these resources represent the costs to each party who engages in a health promotion activity, the benefits to each should also be acknowledged in the development of a marketing plan. For example, people who become active in health promotion programs report such benefits as a better quality of life, higher self-esteem, a general feeling of well-being, better self-image, and more social contacts.[11],[12] Health promotion agencies benefit from offering such programs by being able to meet their organizational goals, increasing their probability of funding from various external sources, and/or conducting more research in the field. However, seldom are these costs and benefits explicitly acknowledged by health education professionals, and rarely are intervention efforts viewed in terms of an exchange process. Rather programs are promoted to the target group with the express interest to minimize monetary costs to them and with only cursory attention given to promotion of the benefits. Two fallacies are evident in this approach: (1) consumer costs are construed only in economic terms, and (2) there is no recognition of the role of the exchange process in utilizing health programs. Public health professionals need to be more attentive to the resource exchange that is inherent in idea dissemination, product use and service delivery and seek to maximize the benefits to both parties rather than attempt only to reduce the costs to one. Later, we discuss incentives and their role in enhancing the exchange process.

Audience Analysis and Segmentation

Audience analysis and the segmentation of a target market into meaningful subgroups is a direct expression of the consumer orientation philosophy. The intent of audience analysis is to identify its needs, document the perceived costs and benefits of addressing the needs, and formulate a program that addresses the needs in the most cost-beneficial manner to both the consumer and the agency. Audience segmentation has two major goals: (1) define homogeneous subgroups for message and product design purposes, and (2) identify segments that will target distribution and communication channel strategies. These segmentation variables include, but are not limited to, geography (region, county, census tract), demography (age, gender, family size, occupation, race, social class), social structure (worksites, churches, voluntary agencies, families, legislative bodies), and psychography (lifestyle, personality, level of readiness for change, identified need — e.g., smokers, channels of communication).[6],[7],[13] Although in theory there are as many segments of an audience as there are individuals or social organizations who constitute the audience, each segment should be relatively homogeneous with respect to certain variables and likely to react differently to a message than other segments. In addition, each segment should be sufficiently large and important enough to justify the allocation of resources to it, should suggest a different marketing mix for the particular product or service, and should be able to be reached efficiently by the agency.[8]

Various direct and indirect methods exist for audience analysis and segmentation. Direct methods include random sampling surveys, observational techniques, questionnaires, and qualitative methods such as personal interviews or focus groups. Indirect methods, which unfortunately are those most often available and affordable by health agencies, include archival methods (e.g., census data, Chamber of Commerce reports) and use of secondary reference material that are based on other sampling populations (e.g., U.S. food consumption patterns, marketing surveys, national polls).[14] However, even these less precise data are underemployed by many health promotion programs though, in many instances, they can provide data directly applicable to the targeted health concern. By not seeking out how the audience perceives its needs, and assuming relative homogeneity of the audience — i.e., "They all have the same problem" — health educators ensure that there will be "hard-to-reach" audiences who are not receptive to their messages, products, and services. A thorough delineation of the target audience and specification of discrete segments that may require different "marketing mixes," while introducing additional complexity into the intervention effort, increases the potential reach and effectiveness of the message, product, or service and its receptivity by the target group. Further specification of the characteristics of these segmented groups relevant to the behavior change process (e.g., past experience knowledge, intentions, perceived efficacy) can be pursued through the use of focus groups and other qualitative research methods to aid in designing products that not only reach the intended audience, but are effective in stimulating the desired behavior change.

Formative Research

The adoption of a marketing approach focuses attention on formative research methods as much as on summative ones. A major lesson to be learned from the marketing literature is the indispensability of market and consumer research that tests concepts, message content and design, and potential new products or services before they are widely disseminated. The importance of formative research is reinforced by Manoff, who suggests that message design is the major task of social marketing; without proper execution, it can be social marketing's critical weakness.[9]

Formative research involves the pretesting of ideas, messages, and methods with representatives of the target group(s) *before* implementation. However, given the pressure many agencies are under to field programs, formative methods are often the first casualty — if they ever appeared in the battle plan. Techniques such as focus groups, samples of convenience, intercept interviews, and pilot studies to test new interventions are more often viewed as luxuries rather than the necessities they are, by both health educators and administrators.

The dangers that are posed by the lack of pretesting can range from the often-told stories of programs that were conceptually elegant but impossible to implement, to absolute public relations nightmares, such as when well-intentioned advertisers designed a message that stimulated unneeded publicity and public debate (e.g., a series of public service announcements for the prevention of child abuse that read "See Dick run. See Spot run. See Jane run . . . Daddy's home").

In an arena characterized by lower levels of funding, the importance of formative research cannot be overemphasized. Although budget-minded persons might view the additional costs of such research as frivolous, it will prove to be money well-spent. Not only can such research suggest changes in program content or delivery that will enhance its reach and/or effectiveness, but it can also circumvent a costly and ill-fated intervention before it receives broad exposure.

Channel Analysis

Public health interventions require a variety of channels through which messages, products and services can be delivered to target groups. These channels may range from mass electronic and print media to influential community leaders and program volunteers. Any person, organization or institution having access to a definable population is a potential channel for health communication. Thus, schools, worksites, social organizations, churches, physicians' offices, and various nonprofit agencies can all be viewed as potential channels of communication. Identification of "life path points" — such as laundromats, grocers, restaurants, bus stops — can also uncover potential channels to reach certain audiences. In addition, techniques such as personal sales, public events, outdoor advertising, direct mail, and telemarketing also provide methods to communicate with the audience. To specify which of these channels, singly or in combination, will best serve the needs of the health agency to reach targeted segments of the community is the major task of channel analysis.

Thorough analysis and selection of communication channels not only presupposes a good understanding of what channels the target audience comes into contact with on a regular basis and perceives as being more influential/ important, but also requires attention to the nature of the message, product or service that will be disseminated.[15] It is also important to be cognizant of the point in the behavior change process at which one is aiming the message. Information and persuasive appeals can be effectively transmitted by mass media channels. Yet, when an individual must decide whether or not to adopt the suggested behavior (e.g., quit smoking, cut down on fatty foods), the interpersonal network is often more influential.[16] Therefore, the nurturance of a group of intermediaries, or opinion leaders, is important to reinforce mass communicated messages and move people through the change process. This point underscores the desirability of targeting influential persons (opinion leaders) early in dissemination efforts so that those persons who are perceived by the social network as homophilous, authoritative and credible sources of information can reinforce adoption of new attitudes and behavior.[16]

Channels can differ in a number of other relevant dimensions.[8] Among the more important ones we include are:

- their ability to transmit complex messages
- their medium — visual, auditory, print, electronic
- their costs
- their reach, frequency, and continuity
- the number of intermediaries they require
- their potential for overuse — or the point at which they oversaturate the market and cease being attended to by the target group
- their capability for multiplicative effects (i.e., ability to build on one another)
- their degree of perceived authority/credibility

The orchestration of selected channels to optimize the reach and saturation of an effective behavior change message is an essential ingredient in health marketing campaigns.

Marketing Mix

The core of designing and implementing marketing plans involves the blending of four distinct elements: (a) products, (b) prices, (c) places, and (d) promotion.[6,10] These so-called "4Ps" have been the object of vigorous research activity in the business and commercial sectors but have only recently been discovered by the health promotion field. We will review each of these elements and discuss their applicability to social marketing and health marketing objectives.

Product

A product is typically conceived of as something tangible: a physical entity or service that can be exchanged with a target market. However, social marketing extends the concept of products to include ideas, social causes and behavior changes (e.g., use contraceptives, eat more fiber). As we have already discussed, a major obstacle to effective social marketing is the intangibility of many products that makes it difficult to market to potential consumers. For example, how does one buy a "healthier life?" The challenge is to begin to make these "intangibles" tangible in a way that appeals to the target audience.

In health marketing there is also the need to create a consumer market for health promotion products and services such as self-help smoking cessation kits, group weight loss programs, blood cholesterol screenings, or corporate fitness challenges. However, rather than viewing this task as simply repetition of health promotion messages, thought needs to be given to these messages as "products" as well. For example, production of public service announcements (PSAs) can appear to be rather straightforward, yet a division at the National Cancer Institute is devoted to pretesting such messages.[17] Curricula, and promotional print pieces such as flyers and posters, all can be treated as products: they are the tangible evidence of the agency to which the consumer can respond. The features, quality, styling, brand name and packaging of each of these "products" can have a far-reaching impact on how the agency is perceived by the market and whether or not consumers will be motivated to try a health promotion product.[6] As much attention needs to be given to these products as to the tests of the effectiveness of the change program.

Product line considerations must also be attended to by health marketing professionals. The dimensions of width, depth, and diversity require ongoing monitoring and evaluation to ensure that programming reaches the largest possible segment of the target audience and can still be effectively managed by the agency.[6] For example, width can be thought of as the number of different target behaviors addressed by the product line (e.g., child accident prevention, breast self-examination and alcohol abuse). Depth refers to the number of products that target each risk behavior across a number of different audience segments (e.g., accident prevention programs directed toward children, older siblings, and parents). Product diversity is the variety of programming that is offered to each target group (e.g., safety talks in classrooms, home visits, informational brochures). Each of these areas should be periodically reviewed, and products added, modified or eliminated as consumer behavior dictates.[6] In health promotion efforts, one particular problem that appears to beset program planners is employing group programs as their major, or only, product line. Such an orientation, in our experience, results in interventions that have relatively low participation rates and may be discontinued within several years because of the lack of participants.[3]

Prices

Prices can be thought of in a variety of ways; in addition to economic reasons, there are social, behavioral, psychological, temporal, structural, geographic, and physical reasons for exchanging or not exchanging. The costs, or barriers, to consumer use of health promotion products receive the most attention. However, another distinguishing feature of the social marketing approach is its use of incentives to encourage participation. Incentives can be both real or perceived, tangible or intangible, financial or social, and so on. Much of what has been learned in social learning research is applicable to this area: people are motivated by incentives, especially those that are tangible and occur shortly after the behavior is practiced.[18] The challenge of health marketing is in both reducing barriers/costs of participation and creating incentives that will further engage people in health and behavior change. For instance, designing contests that offer prizes for individuals, teams, and/or organizations that lose the most weight, exercise most frequently in a given span of time, or quit smoking can result in large numbers of people attempting, and succeeding at, risk factor change.[19-22]

Place

Place characteristics, or distribution channels, add another dimension to the marketing mix. Place decisions need to be based on such considerations as the level and quality of service/coverage one wishes to supply (the inverse rule of "More outlets = Greater reach, but lower quality" generally applies), the number and location of distribution points one can reasonably manage, the use and motivation of intermediaries in product delivery (e.g., gatekeepers, volunteers), and the availability of response channels that are compatible with the distribution system through which the target audience can access the product offering (e.g., tear-off coupons on a promotional flyer).[6] Place decisions are facilitated by in-depth channel analysis prior to implementation. Knowledge of where people are likely to encounter messages in their everyday routines — life path points such as banks, shopping malls, airports — as well as where they congregate — churches, worksites, schools, social clubs — can be used in making distribution decisions. Place features have price implications as well; places can increase costs to consumers by their inaccessibility and distance. However, they can also be used as incentives as, for instance, when health screenings are held in conjunction with city-wide events that have "nonhealth" themes.

Promotion

No decision about the promotion of a health product should be made without a clear outline of the objectives of the promotion — who the target audience will be, what effect is sought, and what the optimal reach and frequency should be. Advertising, publicity, personal contact, and attention to creating an environment designed to produce specific cognitive and/or emotional effects on the target group (atmospherics) are specific ways by which promotion goals can be met.[6] Promotion strategy must be clearly tied to the product, its price, the channels for distribution and the intended target group. All too often, we see program "promotion" that involves very little thought given to the other parts of the equation. Promotion is more than awareness-development or public relations. Used properly, promotion can be a major tool to make health promotion products more acceptable to the public and enhance their utilization by the consumer.

Process Tracking

To provide an integrative and control aspect to the marketing of health promotion programs, it is important to have in place a system that tracks the ongoing activities of the agency. This system should be able to meet a number of evaluation purposes simultaneously, but particularly, it should provide longitudinal data for assessing program delivery and program utilization trends. Specific information that can be included in process tracking includes:

- the activity name — e.g., a blood cholesterol promotion
- the date of the activity
- how it was delivered — e.g., televised PSAs
- the reach of the activity — e.g., 25,000 households
- its objective — e.g., promotion, behavior change, training

For program delivery activities, we would also want to know participant characteristics in addition to the above items. A minimum amount of information — age, gender and, if important to the agency, ethnicity — can provide a wealth of data that will enhance both program delivery evaluation and targeting of activities to underrepresented segments of the population. Over the course of a health marketing program, process tracking data can provide a "big picture" of the agency's activities, identify program elements that are either not offered often enough or are underutilized by the target groups, and help establish priorities in program planning and implementation. Without such data, the agency's management will fail to recognize both the strengths and shortcomings of the marketing plan and will be unable to respond to the shifting needs and priorities of the consumer group.

Marketing Management

Although we find that more health professionals are increasingly open to, and often zealous proponents of, the use of marketing principles in health promotion, the fact remains that in health agencies marketing activities are often poorly understood and insufficiently appreciated by administrators. In addition, if marketing is designated in the organizational structure, it is often inappropriately located.[14] This occurs because of several assumptions: (1) marketing connotes manipulation and thus has no place in the health field, (2) it will require more resources than are available which will then constrain programming, (3) audiences should not be segmented because this will lead to even more "under-served" groups, (4) the terms products, prices, distribution systems, etc., sound more appropriate for a business school than for health promotion, (5) all the emphasis on "research" will impede service delivery, (6) agencies rarely have the staff with marketing expertise to guide and implement a marketing plan, and (7) it demands an unacceptable level of planning and action that may be disruptive to the agency and staff.

There is, in both business and nonprofit sectors, the pervasive belief among managers that an organization that adopts the marketing concept will quickly become "marketing-driven." That is, all program decisions will be left to the whims of the consumer — or the marketing director. There are both pros and cons to this argument, but in setting up a marketing plan and structure within an existing agency, care should be exercised that cherished individual and organizational beliefs and behaviors will be blended into the process. In addition, strong reliance on sound health education and behavior change methods must be maintained.

Case: The Pawtucket Heart Health Program "Know Your Cholesterol" Campaign

One of the first community-wide cholesterol awareness and screening campaigns was conducted by PHHP during March and April, 1985.[24] This campaign was conceived of as the first step in introducing to the general public technology that utilized capillary blood samples for rapid total blood cholesterol determinations. Based on national random sampling data of both the general population and physicians which were available during the planning of the campaign, several objectives were formulated. These included:

- Physician education about the causal relationship of blood cholesterol levels and coronary heart disease (CHD), the technology and accuracy of rapid blood cholesterol analysis to be used in screenings, and action levels for either dietary or drug intervention to lower elevated blood cholesterol.
- Increased awareness among the general population of blood cholesterol as a risk factor for CHD.
- Increased number of people knowing their blood cholesterol level (i.e., attending screening, counseling and referral events — SCOREs — sponsored by PHHP).
- Large numbers of people showing reductions in their blood cholesterol level at two-month follow-up measurements.

Audience needs analyses were based primarily on these data. In segmenting the community of Pawtucket, adults were a primary focus (given that across gender and age awareness levels were equivalent in the national samples). Internists, cardiologists, family medicine specialists, and general medicine physicians were especially targeted for direct mail educational packages and grand rounds presentations on blood cholesterol and heart disease at the community hospital as these were the physicians most likely to see and treat people with high blood cholesterol. Middle-aged men who had previous contact with the PHHP were also the focus of a direct mail and telemarketing campaign to attend SCOREs during the campaign period.

Several formative research efforts preceded campaign planning. These included a pilot test of the efficacy of the self-help "Nutrition Kit" in lowering elevated blood cholesterol levels, and pilots of the SCORE protocol at the local hospital.[25]

Among the channels identified to reach the general and segmented publics were print mass media (because the PHHP comparison community is reached by mass electronic media, this channel was not employed); print media distributed through worksites, churches and schools; direct mail; telemarketing; and SCORE delivery at worksites, churches and various community locations identified as major life path points (e.g., grocery stores, St. Patrick's Day Parade, shopping plazas). In mixing the 4Ps, price emerged as an important variable. SCOREs were initially priced at $5.00 per person. This fee covered the costs of materials for both an initial and follow-up measurement. We reasoned that people who had already paid for a second measurement would be more likely to have a follow-up test than if they had to pay for it separately. This pricing strategy also allowed for price reductions/specials (e.g., all men targeted by direct mail and telemarketing efforts received coupons good for $1.00 off the "usual" price).

Promotional strategies included the "kick-off" SCORE at the St. Patrick's Day Parade and six weekly columns in the local newspaper on the diet, blood cholesterol, and CHD relationship that featured specific advice and tips on a heart health eating pattern. The selection of a variety of locations for SCOREs helped ensure that different segments of the Pawtucket population would have access to this service.

The process tracking data from this campaign have been previously reported.[24] Briefly, 39 SCOREs were attended by 1,439 adults, 60% of whom were identified as having elevated blood cholesterol levels. Two months after the campaign, 72.3% of these persons had returned for a second measurement. Nearly 60% of this group had reduced their blood cholesterol level by an average of 29.1 mg/dl. More important than these short-term results has been the integration of the essential components of this campaign into ongoing PHHP intervention activities. This marketing strategy has led to over 10,000 persons having had their blood cholesterol measured in the subsequent two years, all of whom have received information on how to help themselves make dietary changes to manage elevated levels, and many have subsequently been referred to their physician for more intensive treatment. Interestingly, a recent survey of local physicians' attitudes and practice towards treating elevated blood cholesterol found them to be more aggressive in initiating either diet or drug therapy than either their colleagues in a neighboring community or those who participated in a national sampling of physicians conducted contemporaneously with our own. A major reason cited by Pawtucket physicians for changing their practice was patient requests for blood cholesterol measurements and/or dietary information.[26] One could conclude from these observations that an informed marketplace can, in fact, influence changes in physicians' treatment of elevated blood cholesterol levels when coordinated through campaigns and strategic follow-up activities.

Case: The Stanford Five-City Project Smokers' Challenge II

In February, 1983, the FCP launched a quit smoking contest after conducting a smoking cessation television series and a self-help print campaign. Smokers' motivations to quit and their preferred methods of quitting were gathered from our community survey data. From these data, and with analyses of the demographic profiles of participants in group programs, we decided to reach smokers who were not highly motivated to quit, to try to get more men into the program, and to use incentives in the program. Several objectives were formulated for this 6-week quit smoking contest. These included:

- achieving broad awareness of the contest in the general population
- recruiting a large number of smokers to sign up for the contest
- encouraging over 50% of the participating smokers to use community resources to quit
- achieving a quit rate at the end of the contest that was greater than other minimal contact programs (more than 20%)
- providing those quitters with the skills to remain nonsmokers for one year.

The audience needs analysis then led us to establish moderately motivated male smokers as the target audience for the program and to utilize incentives to recruit them to the program and to encourage compliance with quit smoking advice. Several phases of formative evaluation were carried out to refine the contest strategy and promotion. To decide upon a title for the contest and the types of appeal for the promotional materials, smokers at local bars and after work gatherings were shown titles and sample ads and interviewed about the effectiveness of these materials. The results of these informal interviews yielded a contest called "Smokers' Challenge;" an appeal to smokers only; and promotional materials focused on the title first, the prize second and the contest information third.

Smokers responding to a community random phone survey ($n = 97$) were asked what type of incentive (if any) would motivate them to participate in the contest. They were presented with the option of a trip to a local urban area, a color television set, and a car. The rate of a positive response to each alternative corresponded to the size of the prize or the incentive (trip 25%, television set 47%, car 67%). All prizes were donated by community groups; however, we were unable to obtain a car as the grand prize. Instead we were able to get a trip to Hawaii for two. We reasoned that the price of this prize was somewhat between the price of a car and a television set in price and would suffice as an adequate incentive.

Based on past experience and community population data on media use patterns we selected television, newspaper, libraries, worksites, schools, stores, and physicians' offices as the primary channels for promoting the contest. In addition, the community organization strategy of co-sponsorship was used to encourage the TV station to expand the frequency and intensity of message dissemination beyond traditional PSA play. Messages produced by the TV station were played 82 times in one month.

Price in the overall marketing mix included program cost, energy costs to sign up, and psychological costs (coping with urges, relapse prevention etc.). The overall goal of the price analysis was to not impose barriers to participate in the contest for smokers who were moderately interested in quitting. Since large scale recruitment and participation was crucial to the success of the program, we decided to remove financial and access barriers in the recruitment (we could only recruit at a limited number of distribution sites if fees were charged for participating in the contest) and to advertise community quit smoking programs that either were free or that charged a fee in the participation phase of the contest.

As presented in a published report,[22] only some of the outcome objectives were achieved; the results of a random phone population survey indicated that approximately 60% of the community were aware of the program, 501 smokers signed up for the program, more women (55%) than men were recruited (though the proportion of men was higher than other FCP group and self-help programs in the community), only a few signed up for community programs (11 groups, 22% self-help materials), 45% quit for a short time, and 22% quit with a one year maintenance rate of 15%.

From analysis of the quit data, process tracking of the contest, and additional focus group discussions, it was decided that the promotion of the contest had been effective. It was also found that the quitting materials may not have appealed to the smokers who participated, that these quitting materials were sometimes not available at the contest sign-up locations, and that participating smokers needed more support to stay quit. Revisions were made based on our experiences with the Smokers' Challenge I contest:

- New quitting materials were developed that were more directive, and gave smokers a day-by-day set of guidelines for quitting in 12 days. This revised self-help program was supported by a 12-day radio show that reinforced the principles in the booklet. Based on smokers' stated preference for "cold turkey" approaches to quitting, this new guide was titled "Cool Turkey."

- These new materials were the only quitting approach advertised in the recruitment materials: they were mailed to all participants requesting them, thus improving access to quitting information.

- The contest was expanded from six weeks to three months. Smokers could earn chances for both the final prize and for smaller prizes if they sent in monthly "quit cards."

A second Smokers Challenge contest attracted 588 smokers. Forty-five percent of entrants were male, 40% had less than a high school education (similar to the first contest), over 70% of participants signed up for the "Cold Turkey" booklet, 30% sent in the quit cards at the end of the contest, and a survey follow-up at three months after the contest with an alveolar carbon monoxide assessment on 20 entrants revealed a 30% quit rate. We established that access to quitting information was important to use and quit rates, and that a longer contest — while much more difficult to manage — yielded improved short-term and interim results. We also saw that the demographics of contest participants were strikingly stable across both challenges. The new marketing mix with a revised product illustrates that process tracking during events and outcome evaluation are crucial to strategy refinement and goal readjustment.

Limits of Social Marketing

Given the many strengths and strategies provided by adopting social marketing principles for public health change, it is important to note that social marketing is not a panacea for many of the problems that beset health educators, planners, agencies, and policy makers. Several years ago, Bloom and Novelli[14] outlined nine areas of problems and challenges that face the individual or organization attempting to apply social marketing principles. The areas highlighted by them included problems in market analyses, market segmentation, product strategy, positioning strategy, pricing strategy, channel strategy, communications strategy, organizational design and planning, and evaluation. The reader is referred to their article for a more complete review of their concerns.

Manoff[9] also noted that there are a variety of socio-economic constraints that must be addressed by social marketers. His list includes such factors as antithetical marketing practices by other concerns, faddist and unhealthful lifestyles, lack of supportive public policies, a lack of consensus among health authorities (either on what the problem is or what to do about it), and a lack of coordination of various health agencies' efforts.

Social marketing has also been decried as another form of "blaming the victim" — that is, assigning the cause of health problems to individuals and focusing all attempts at change on individual-based strategies. However, this is a very narrow conceptualization of the purview of social marketing and, as indicated by Manoff, there are many socio-economic and environmental concerns that can be addressed, and should be addressed, by social marketers in marketing public health.

Discussions of marketing also raise ethical questions such as "What are we selling?", "Who are we selling it to?", "How are we selling it?", and "Whose side are we on?" These questions, and many other issues about "the business of health promotion" have been addressed in detail by others.[23] We believe that it is important for health marketers to ask themselves these tough questions, and be prepared to identify the limits of their knowledge and expertise. While social marketing practices can certainly be usurped in ways counter to ethical and professional sensibilities, it is equally likely that social marketing practices can be employed by persons with limited knowledge, appreciation and respect for what they can and cannot achieve.

Conclusion

What is the incentive for marketing health — rather than promoting it? Essentially, from our experience we believe that a well-functioning marketing operation can provide a manager/administrator with a level of analysis, planning, implementation, and control of agency operations that can lead to more effective and efficient use of resources and improved consumer satisfaction. Once staff members understand marketing concepts, organizational objectives, and their role in the organization from a marketing perspective — and act on this information on a daily basis — they can formulate programs that are strategically designed to satisfy organizational goals. Health marketing has the potential of reaching the largest possible group of people at the least cost with the most effective, consumer-satisfying program. The availability of market research helps identify population needs and preferences. Audience analysis allows the agency to specify the goals of the program, identify relevant target audiences, and refine the proposed behavior changes. Formative research can be utilized to define and test the proposed change strategies, further elaborate audience needs and possible points of resistance to the proposed strategies, and guard against the misappropriation of resources to ineffective or unattractive products. Channel analyses can help formulate cost-effective ways to reach the target audience. Attention to the 4Ps in intervention planning and implementation, and the addition of a process tracking system that can provide basic information on activities and program participants, provide methods that can optimize the efficiency of the entire project and feed back valuable data that can be used to reposition products and fine-tune the change strategy. Finally, carefully controlled outcome studies of program effectiveness can provide the bottom-line test as to whether the marketing plan is, in fact, achieving its objectives and resulting in a healthier population.

References

[1] Ward, G.W. 1984. The National High Blood Pressure Education Program: A description of its utility as a generic program model. *Health Education Quarterly* 11:225-42.

[2] Myer, A. J., Maccoby, N., and Farquhar, J. W. 1977. The role of opinion leadership in a cardiovascular health education campaign. In B.D. Ruben (ed.), *Communication Yearbook I.* New Brunswick, NJ: Transaction Books.

[3] Lefebvre, R. C., Harden, E.A., Rakowski, W., Lasater, T. M., and Carleton, R. A. 1987. Characteristics of participants in community health promotion programs: Four-year results. *AJPH* 77:1342-44.

[4] Lefebvre R. C., Lasater, T. M., Carleton, R. A., and Peterson, G. 1987. Theory and delivery of health programming in the community: The Pawtucket Heart Health Program. *Preventive Medicine* 16:80-95.

[5] Farquhar, J. W., Fortmann, S. P., Maccoby, N., Haskell, W. L., Williams, P. T., Flora, J. A., Taylor C. B., Brown, Jr., B. W., Solomon, D. S., and Hulley, S. B. 1985. The Stanford Five-City Project: Design and methods. *American Journal Epid* 122:323-34.

[6] Kotler, P. 1975. *Marketing for nonprofit organizations.* Englewood Cliffs, NJ: Prentice-Hall.

[7] Novelli, W. D. 1984. Developing marketing programs. In Frederickson, L. W., Solomon, L. J., and Brehony, K. A. (eds.), *Marketing health behavior: Principles, techniques and applications.* New York: Plenum.

[8] Fine, S. H. 1981. *The marketing of ideas and social issues.* New York: Praeger.

[9] Manoff, R. K. 1985. *Social marketing.* New York: Praeger.

[10] Kotler, P., and Zaltman, G. 1971. Social marketing: An approach to planned social change. *J Marketing* 35:3-12.

[11] Blair, S. N., Smith, M., Collingwood, T. R., Reynolds, R., Prentice, M. C., and Sterlin, C. L. 1986. Health education for educators: Impact on absenteeism. *Preventive Medicine* 15:166-75.

[12] Green, L. W., Wilson, A. L., and Lovato, C. Y. 1986. What changes can health promotion achieve and how long do these changes last? The trade-offs between expediency and durability. *Preventive Medicine* 15:508-21.

[13] Murphy, P. E. 1984. Analyzing markets. In Frederickson, L. W., Solomon, L. J., and Brehony, K. A. (eds.), *Marketing health behavior: Principles, techniques and applications.* New York: Plenum.

[14] Bloom, P. N., and Novelli, W. D. 1981. Problems and challenges of social marketing. *J Marketing* 45:79-88.

[15] Lefebvre, R. C., Harden, E. A., and Zompa, B. 1988. The Pawtucket Heart Health Program: Social marketing to promote community health. *Rhode Island Medical Journal* 71:27-30.

[16] Rogers, E. M. 1983. *Diffusion of Innovations* (3rd ed.). New York: Free Press.

[17] U.S. Department of Health and Human Services. 1984. *Pretesting in health communications* (NIH Publication No. 84-1493. Bethesda, MD: National Cancer Institute).

[18] Bandura, A. 1977. *Social learning theory.* Englewood Cliffs, NJ: Prentice-Hall.

[19] Elder, J. P., McGraw, S. A., Rodrigues, A., Lasater, T. M., Ferreira, A., Kendall, L., Peterson, G. S., and Carleton, R. A. 1987. Evaluation of two community-wide smoking cessation contests. *Preventive Medicine* 16:221-34.

[20] Nelson, D. J., Sennett, L., Lefebvre, R. C., Loiselle, L., McClements, L., and Carleton, R. A. 1987. A campaign strategy for weight loss at worksites. *Health Education Research: Theory and Practice* 2:27-31.

[21] Altman, D. G., Flora, J. A., Fortman, S. P., and Farquhar, J. W. 1987. The cost-effectiveness of three smoking cessation programs, *AJPH* 77:162-65.

[22] King, A. C., Flora, J. A., Fortmann, S. P., and Taylor, C. B. 1987. Smokers' challenge: Immediate and long-term findings of a community smoking cessation contest. *AJPH* 77:1341-42.

[23] McLeroy, K. R., Gottlieb, N. H., and Burdine, J. N. 1987. The business of health promotion: Ethical issues and professional responsibilities. *Health Education Quarterly* 14:91-109.

[24] Lefebvre, R. C., Peterson, G. S., McGraw, S. A., Lasater, T. M., Sennett, L., Kendall, L., and Carleton, R. A. 1986. Community intervention to lower blood cholesterol: The "Know Your Cholesterol" campaign in Pawtucket, Rhode Island. *Health Education Q* 13:117-29.

[25] Peterson, G. S., Lefebvre, R. C., Ferreira A., Sennett, L., Lazieh, M., and Carleton, R. A. 1986. Strategies for cholesterol lowering at the worksite. *J Nutr Education* 18:S54-S57.

[26] Block, L. W., Banspach, S. W., Gans, K., Harris, C., Lasater, T. M., Lefebvre, R. C., and Carleton, R. A. In press. Impact of public education and continuing medical education on physician attitudes and behavior concerning cholesterol. *American Journal of Preventive Medicine.*